Compulsive Sexual B

Compulsive Sexual Behaviours offers a unique approach to the struggles people face with their out-of-control sexual behaviours.

This comprehensive guide is deeply rooted in the science of sexology and psychotherapy, demonstrating why it is time to re-think the reductive concept of 'sex addiction' and move towards a more modern age of evidence-based, pluralistic and sex-positive psychotherapy. It is an important manual for ethical, safe and efficient treatment within a humanistic and relational philosophy.

This book will be an important guide in helping clients stop their compulsive sexual behaviours as well as for therapists to self-reflect on their own morals and ethics so that they can be prepared to explore their clients' erotic mind.

Silva Neves is a COSRT accredited and UKCP registered psychotherapist, specialising in sexology, relationships and trauma. He is a course director for CICS (Contemporary Institute of Clinical Sexology), an international speaker and an editorial board member of the leading journal *Sex and Relationship Therapy*.

Compulsive Sexual Behaviours

A Psycho-Sexual Treatment Guide for Clinicians

Silva Neves

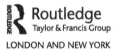

Routledge
Taylor & Francis Group

LONDON AND NEW YORK

First published 2021
by Routledge
2 Park Square, Milton Park, Abingdon, Oxon OX14 4RN

and by Routledge
605 Third Avenue, New York, NY 10158

Routledge is an imprint of the Taylor & Francis Group, an informa business

British Library Cataloguing-in-Publication Data
A catalogue record for this book is available from the British Library

Library of Congress Cataloging-in-Publication Data
Names: Neves, Silva, author.
Title: Compulsive sexual behaviours : a psycho-sexual treatment guide for clinicians / Silva Neves.
Description: Abingdon, Oxon ; New York, NY : Routledge, 2021. |
Includes bibliographical references and index. |
Identifiers: LCCN 2020053484 (print) | LCCN 2020053485 (ebook) |
ISBN 9780367465506 (hardback) | ISBN 9780367465483 (paperback) |
ISBN 9781003029502 (ebook)
Subjects: LCSH: Sex addiction. | Sex addiction--Treatment.
Classification: LCC RC560.S43 N48 2021 (print) | LCC RC560.S43
(ebook) | DDC 616.85/833--dc23
LC record available at https://lccn.loc.gov/2020053484
LC ebook record available at https://lccn.loc.gov/2020053485

ISBN: 978-0-367-46550-6 (hbk)
ISBN: 978-0-367-46548-3 (pbk)
ISBN: 978-1-003-02950-2 (ebk)

Typeset in Times New Roman
by MPS Limited, Dehradun

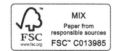
MIX
Paper from
responsible sources
FSC   FSC™ C013985
www.fsc.org

Printed in the United Kingdom
by Henry Ling Limited

Contents

Preface

It would be safe to say that the concepts of sex and porn addiction are controversial in the field of psychotherapy. The debate is strongly polarised between professionals who assert that sex and porn addictions exist and those that as vociferously state that sex and pornography are not addictive. No-one refutes that clients access therapy for help with sexual behaviours that they feel they have no control over. The issue is how these client experiences are conceptualised and how the clinical formulation informs treatment.

After years of study and clinical practice with the presenting issue of unwanted sexual behaviours, Silva Neves is clear that the sex addiction approach is inadequate. In this much needed book he refocuses the therapist to explore the client's erotic template and the drivers behind their compulsivity, rather than on behavioural prevention. He offers a trauma informed, three phase treatment approach to the resolution of compulsivity, that honours the unique sexuality and sexual expression of the client. Crucially, he brings clarity to the conflation between sexual compulsivity and sex offending that is often made in sex addiction discourses.

This book is a generous sharing of Silva's experience with the evident intention to help its reader to provide a sexology informed, non-shaming service to clients presenting with the complex experience of sexual compulsivity. It is research based, contemporary, inclusive and pluralistic. It is a must read for all professionals working with the themes of sex, relationships, addiction and compulsion.

Julie Sale
Director of The Contemporary Institute of Clinical Sexology, COSRT
Senior Accredited Sex and Relationship Therapist and Supervisor, UKCP
Registered and Accredited Psychotherapist

Acknowledgments

First of all, I would like to thank my colleague and friend who took the hard job of being my editor for this book, Julie Sale. Her warmth, her love for the profession and her focus were great gifts to me. Without her, this book will have never been published.

I would like to warmly thank my clinical supervisor Dominic Davies who is the leading clinician in gender, sexuality and relationship diversity in the UK. His wisdom and his generosity in sharing his professional connections are the seeds of my flourishing into writing this book.

I would like to thank my other clinical supervisors, Jean Miller and Dr Manda Holmshaw who have been consistent sources of support in my professional growth. I'm also grateful for Dr Douglas Braun-Harvey who facilitated a UK-based group supervision which was very helpful at the genesis of this book. I cannot forget clinical supervisors of the past; Dr Jacob Jacobson was the first one who alerted me to the limitations of the 'sex addiction' framework, when I was a young therapist learning about this presentation.

I would like to thank my wonderful colleagues, some of whom I am proud to call my friends, who are all champions in sexology, gender, sexuality and relationship diversity. One way or another, they have influenced me and contributed to this book: Kate Moyle, Dr Roberta Babb, Lohani Noor, Dr Meg-John Barker, Dr Joe Kort, Dr David Ley, Dr Nicole Prause, Remziye Kunelaki, Dr Francesca Tripoli, Dr Evie Kirana, Dr Filippo Nimbi.

I would like to thank Babette Rothschild, one of the world leading experts in trauma. I'm so lucky to have benefited from her teachings. When she first met me, she probably never imagined she would be cited in a book on compulsive sexual behaviours, but there it is.

I'm grateful to Jack Morin, a clinician I never had the pleasure to meet but a real pioneer in sexology.

I would like to thank COSRT (College Of Sexual and Relationship Therapists) for being my professional home. I'm privileged to have such a wonderful professional network.

Last, but not least, I would like to thank my husband Dr James Rafferty who spent many weekends entertaining himself whilst I wrote this book. His consistent patience, love and radical acceptance is my secure base.

Introduction

Writing this book has been a long journey. Let me tell you about the beginning. I grew up in France. Two cultural points of being French are engrained in my psyche from which I see the world. The first one is pleasure. French people love taking their time for their pleasure unapologetically, especially the pleasure of food. The second is the value of secularism. The Age of Enlightenment in the 17th century was largely influenced by French thinking, whereby scientific evidence took priority over ideology. You will see these personal cultural references throughout this book. I identify as a cis-gay man. The history of my LGBTQ+ community is one that had been harmed and traumatised with erroneous medical and psychiatric diagnosis on sexual behaviours. I am too aware that words used in clinical settings are important because they can hurt, they can shame, they can prompt suicide. They can also be powerfully healing.

After my core integrative psychotherapeutic training, I did a further postgraduate training in psychosexual and relationship therapy. After that, I became interested in 'sex addiction' mostly because I found it curious that this specialist field paid so little attention to sexology. I spent a number of years following the 'sex addiction' model because there simply weren't any trainings available that was psychosexually oriented. But after a while, I realised that much of my clinical times with clients was to help them not 'relapse', yet, 'relapse' was so common. I thought I didn't have the talent for working with such population. I decided to leave the 'sex addiction' clinic I was working for at the time. But my curiosity helping these clients battling with their sexual compulsivity only grew. By then, I was doing my thing, in my own consulting room, feeling like a rogue, because I was on my own working with my clients with good old-fashioned psychotherapy. I felt like a fraud. I felt alone in this. Along the way in my journey, I completed a diploma in eating disorders, and then I had a lightbulb moment. Treating the impulse control for binge eating could be adapted for treating sexual compulsivity. With the help of my clinical supervisor, I began to notice that there were other voices, those of sexologists, neuroscientists, scientific researchers worldwide concurring with my clinical experience. I had to be truly far away from the 'sex addiction' noise to properly hear those voices. But once I heard them, I knew I had found a clinical community that actually made sense to me. I am grateful to all my colleagues who helped me along the way in my understanding of such a complex clinical presentation. This book is my small contribution for my peers, to say thank you, and hopefully, it will encourage more clinicians to re-think the conceptualisation of 'sex addiction' so that more people can benefit from a treatment that is evidenced-based.

Part I

Understanding compulsive sexual behaviours

Chapter 1

A pluralistic perspective beyond the addiction thinking

The topic of 'sex addiction' is still a contentious debate amongst professionals. Whilst the 'sex addiction' thinking dominated the profession for many years, a growing number of clinicians are moving away from that conceptualisation as there is now a large body of clinical evidence that supports sexual compulsivity to be quite a different phenomenon (Ley, 2012; Magnanti, 2012; Bering, 2013; Donaghue, 2015; Braun-Harvey and Vigorito, 2016). As research and critical thinking goes on, the limitations of the addiction-focused model are becoming more evident. Over many years of working with clients presenting with sexual compulsivity, and studying the topic in depth, I have come to the conclusion that a pluralistic approach is essential for an effective and ethical treatment, as indicated by Cooper and McLeod:

> The essence of this approach is the assumption that different clients may want different things from counselling and psychotherapy at different points in time (2011, p. 13).

It requires an understanding of multiple psychotherapeutic orientations in order to meet the needs of clients in the here-and-now. I draw my interventions from the field of sexology and various psychotherapy modalities. In my opinion, this approach has more to offer than the single framework of addiction.

It does matter what we call it

Many therapists are confused with the terms addiction and compulsivity. Some think they are the same. Some think it doesn't matter what you call it. Some say that if a behaviour is out of control then it is an addiction. All of these thoughts are reductive and they serve the purpose of avoiding being challenged. Before I go on with the definitions and explain the distinct differences, let me tell you first that, yes, it does matter what you call it because it determines the treatment you offer to clients. A cough may be a common cold, lung cancer or a speck of dust stuck in your throat. It certainly matters what the cough is to get the right treatment. The psychotherapy field should uphold the same rigorous approach as the medical profession; a failure to do so is negligence, in my opinion.

Addiction

Addiction is a complex pathology understood in the context of substances introduced in the body that creates physiological and psychological consequences. The Diagnostic and Statistical Manual of Mental Disorders (DSM-5) classifies the pathology under 'Substance Use Disorders' with the following criteria:

1. Impaired control: unsuccessful attempts to reduce or stop using the substance. Spending a lot of time obtaining, using and recovering from the substance. Intense urge to take the substance, called cravings.
2. Social impairment: failure to meet life's obligations because of the substance use. Continued use of the substance despite negative consequences. Social activities stop or are avoided in order to continue using the substance.
3. Risky use: using the substance in a dangerous way. Unable to stop using it even when there are clear ongoing physical and psychological problems.
4. Tolerance: needs an increased dose to achieve the desired effect.
5. Withdrawal: a physical discomfort when the level of substance reduces in the blood and tissue.

It is easy to mistake sexual compulsivity for an addiction because we often hear clients struggling with impaired control and, sometimes, but not always, social impairment. However, in sexual behaviours, the elements of risky use, tolerance and withdrawal are not present.

Risky use: there is a risk of contracting a sexually transmitted infection, which is damaging, but it will not kill people. Some clients may put themselves in risky situations when engaging in compulsive sex, although it is not common or frequent.

Tolerance: implies that the sexual behaviour has to be pleasurable to start with and then stops being pleasurable, so the person needs to do more of it to achieve the same effect. This is one of the major criteria of addiction that is not present in sexual behaviours. Sexual pleasure never stops being pleasurable and people don't need to have more sex to achieve the same pleasure. People sometimes report not feeling pleasure from their compulsive sexual behaviours. It is not because they have become desensitised to it and need more of it, it is because they have dissociated from it, which is a big difference. People mindlessly eating their favourite cheese may not feel the pleasure of the taste in that moment, but they will continue to have the same enjoyment of their cheese when they eat it mindfully.

Withdrawal: is also another major criterion that has never been observed in sexual behaviours because our body is naturally designed to sustain the brain chemicals involved in the pleasure experience of sex and orgasms.

The DSM-5 explains the phenomenon of craving as:

> an intense desire or urge for the drug that may occur at any time but is more likely when in an environment where the drug previously was obtained or used (2013, p. 483).

Addiction experts call the association of an environment with the intense urge 'cue reactivity'. This is quite confusing for addiction professionals who have no training in sexology because they can mistake the pathological addiction of cue reactivity with the normative one of sexual desire and arousal. Sexual stimuli naturally bring sexual arousal in a non-pathological way.

Prominent addiction expert Gabor Maté defines addiction more broadly incorporating 'behavioural addiction', also called 'process addiction':

> Addiction is any repeated behaviour, substance-related or not, in which a person feels compelled to persist, regardless of its negative impact on his life and the lives of others (2018, p. 128).

Neuroscientist Marc Lewis refers to sex as an addiction too but argues that addictions should not be conceptualised as a disease:

> If addiction is a disease, then so, apparently, is love (2015, p. 168).

Lewis makes the analogy of addiction as *'false advertising'*:

> The striatum responds with eager anticipation to the glitter bestowed by our wishes and fantasies. But the high is never as good as promised and, worse, it doesn't last (2015, p. 171).

The American Psychiatric Association, however, excludes 'sex addiction' and 'behavioural addiction' from the DSM-5:

> groups of repetitive behaviors, which some term behavioral addiction, with such subcategories as "sex addiction", "exercise addiction", or "shopping addiction", are not included because at this time there is insufficient peer-reviewed evidence to establish the diagnostic criteria and course descriptions needed to identify these behaviors as mental disorders (2013, p. 481).

Neuroscientists who are sex researchers concur with the DSM-5:

> To date, research on the effects of sex on glutamate function and its modulation of dopamine pathways is scarce. Sex is primary reward, with unique peripheral representation. Engagement in sex is positively associated with health and life satisfaction. Sex does not allow for supraphysiological stimulation (Prause et al., 2017).

The American Association of Sexuality Educators, Counselors and Therapists (AASECT) made a clear statement on their website regarding 'sex addiction':

> it is the position of AASECT that linking problems related to sexual urges, thoughts or behaviors to a porn/sexual addiction process cannot be advanced by AASECT as a standard of practice for sexuality education delivery, counseling or therapy.

The World Health Organisation (WHO) and the International Classification of Disease (ICD-11) classified the condition as 'Compulsive Sexual Behaviour Disorder' (CSBD), under the impulse control category, not addiction. The Medical Services Advisory Committee, whose role it is to advise WHO in the development of the ICD-11, states:

> materials in the ICD-11 make very clear that CSBD is not intended to be interchangeable with sex addiction, but rather is a substantially different diagnostic framework

Compulsivity and impulsivity

Berlin and Hollander (2008) summarise impulsivity as a:

> tendency to act prematurely and without foresight for the purpose to increase arousal.

They define compulsivity as:

> a tendency to repeat the same, often purposeless acts, which are sometimes associated with undesirable consequences for the purpose of relief of tension.

A compulsive behaviour aims to reduce unpleasant emotions. People with compulsivity are fully aware that their behaviours are irrational because they do not have any links to the unpleasant emotions they are trying to reduce, yet, they can't stop the behaviours. For example, someone compulsively washing their hands knows that they won't be able to irradicate germs. Someone compulsively eating biscuits knows that the biscuits won't fix their anxiety. But the stress and anxiety that these people feel is relieved temporarily at the moment of the compulsive behaviour. Crucially, there is no pleasure experienced with compulsive behaviours. We can understand compulsive sexual behaviours' undercurrent purpose as both an attempt to increase arousal as well as relieving tension. Both are good strategies to manage emotional disturbances if the client doesn't have other strategies for emotional resilience. Increasing arousal and relieving tension can also be a normal function of sex that doesn't necessarily respond to emotional disturbances.

In contrast, some people find impulsivity exciting because they enjoy the thrill despite the possible negative consequences. For example the impulse of '*I might get caught having sex in the woods*' may produce a thrill-seeking excitement. In other words, impulsivity is an active going towards pleasure and compulsivity is an active moving away from unpleasant emotions. It is important to consider the function of impulsivity and compulsivity with each client to help them understand how they can regulate them better, like driving a car, with a consistent balance between acceleration and braking.

However, both the pathology of addiction and the understanding of compulsivity assume that sex stops feeling good. This is where the two models fail to fully describe people's sexual behaviour problems. It is very rare to meet someone who likes sex experiencing no pleasure from it.

The problems with the 'sex addiction' approach

As mentioned earlier, what we call it determines the treatment. 'Sex addiction' therapists are congruent with their beliefs and their treatment. The typical addiction treatment primarily focuses on stopping behaviours and avoiding 'triggers'. In the 'sex addiction' thinking, it translates into avoiding anything that has the potential of being sexual or arousing: attractive people, posters showing models in bikinis, sexual scenes on television or movies, sexual jokes, any sexual stimuli, including sexual fantasies!

> The simplest and most effective strategy is simply to look away (...) Other strategies include making sure you're facing the wall in public places so you're less likely to notice people or scan on the off chance (Hall, 2019, p. 146).

These types of typical addiction strategies are problematic because they encourage clients to be erotically avoidant, which is not a sustainable outcome. Being that avoidant makes for a pretty miserable life of deprivation; it's like being on a spinach diet, with no dressing.

Although there have never been any reports of death from orgasm overdose, 'sex addiction' professionals try very hard to apply the addiction definition to sex, making clients believe that there is a tolerance to these behaviours which escalate to unmanageable levels. The 'sex addiction' field tries to instil fear of the addiction by discussing the dangers of contracting sexually-transmitted infections or the sexual behaviours escalating to illegal territory, confusing sexual compulsivity with sexual offending, which are, in fact, two distinctly different clinical presentations. Carnes (2001) erroneously classifies sexual offending under what he calls the '*Level 3*' of 'sex addiction'. Telling people that sexual compulsivity can lead to sexual assault is gross misinformation and does a great disservice to the public. In fact, the field of 'sex addiction' was highly criticised for offering an excuse for serious criminal behaviours when Harvey Weinstein booked himself into a 'sex addiction' clinic after being accused of multiple sexual assaults.

Therapists trained in 'sex addiction' routinely recommend 12-step programmes such as Sex Addict Anonymous (SAA) or Sex and Love Addicts Anonymous (SLAA). Reading the Sex Addicts Anonymous book raises immediate concerns from a sex therapist's perspective. The Sex Addicts Anonymous book (2005), which proudly confirms that it is only anecdotal, nevertheless makes its statement that 'sex addiction' is a progressive '*disease*', stating clearly that its goal is '*sexual sobriety*'. These 12-step programmes have a long list of sexual behaviours they think are 'unhealthy', encouraging their followers to fear normative sexual behaviours by putting them in the same category as illegal non-consensual behaviours. At the same time, these programmes remain pretty vague about what they describe as 'healthy' sex although I imagine it is safe to assume the Fellowship would deem marital, heterosexual, monogamous, vanilla sex to be the gold standard. If we follow its guidance, it means that we should have heteronormative sex between two people in a committed relationship, looking lovingly into each other's eyes, with a frequency of … not too much. This is indeed the description of great sex for some people, but definitely not optimum for many others.

The Sex Addicts book proclaims to be non-religious, yet it encourages its followers to avoid being personally responsible and to rely on the external '*Higher Power*' instead. 12-step programmes rely on their followers to never leave their community in order to keep existing, just like a religion. The word '*God*' is mentioned numerous times in the book. The authors call people who are reluctant to enter the programme 'in denial', but I think it is they who are in denial.

Because of the many problematic teachings of Sex Addicts Anonymous, I challenge 'sex addiction' therapists who call themselves 'sex-positive' and 'integrative' and yet routinely recommend a SAA or SLAA 12-step programme. I fail to see how any therapy professionals can be both 'sex-positive' and promote SAA or SLAA, unless they are holding the view that the only 'positive' sex is monogamous and heterosexual.

A study by Hartmann (2020) reveals that the anti-masturbation movement NoFap is part of a manosphere promoting harmful values on masculinity and misogyny that do not match the values of psychotherapy and sexology. Do your own research before recommending such groups to clients. If your training organisation, supervisor or a 'sex addiction' expert promotes it, beware, it does not mean it is good!

In summary, I think the 'sex addiction' approach is not appropriate because it is sex-negative and pleasure-negative. It is incongruent with the scientific knowledge on human sexuality. There is a great risk of sexual shaming, and there is a great risk of harming clients. I do not use the word 'harm' lightly. As a psychotherapist specialised in sex and trauma, I have seen many people coming to me for help with recovering from the trauma of their 'sex addiction' treatment. They often report feeling worse about themselves and their sexuality. They do not speak up about it because of their intense shame induced by such treatment.

The non-pathological psychosexual approach with sexual compulsivity

The compulsivity model does not completely describe the clinical presentations of compulsive sexual behaviours. However, it does offer us evidence-based treatment protocols, unlike the 'sex addiction' approach. A central concept of compulsivity treatment is the use of Exposure with Response Prevention (Lindsay et al., 1997; Foa et al., 1980), a strategy helping clients to confront their fears whilst not engaging in their compulsions. The sexual compulsivity model actively discourages avoiding sexual cues or stopping behaviours; in fact, it is focused on helping clients face and manage sexual stimuli, in other words, it is helping clients become more erotically aware rather than erotically avoidant. However, the compulsivity approach is not enough in itself, because therapists need to have a robust understanding of sexology so that they can guide clients effectively towards thriving sexually. Whilst the compulsivity approach can be useful in managing sexual stimuli, the psychosexual knowledge will help clients fully own their erotic selves. Rather than the spinach diet, it is sitting at the delicious banquet and enjoying all the food, tasting it properly, taking time with it, like a professional gastronome. This is the philosophy of this book.

My prediction is that the terminology 'sex addiction' will eventually be shelved with the old-fashioned shaming and pathologising terms of misunderstood sexual behaviours, along with 'nymphomania', 'hysteria', and 'homosexuality'. My hope is that the ICD (who has shown to be slow at depathologising sexual behaviours, given that they only took homosexuality off the list of mental health disorders in 1990), may eventually take Compulsive Sexual Behaviours Disorder off the list altogether. These compulsive sexual problems can be understood without the pathology of either addiction or compulsivity, but more as what it is actually likely to be: a strategy that helps people check out from unpleasant emotions by engaging in behaviours that are pleasurable and continue to be pleasurable. In other words, the same type of behaviours as people binging on television, chocolate, exercise, golf, and whatever else to help them manage a stressful life, without calling it a disorder. Interestingly, Galen Fous proposes an alternative term '*Sexual Authenticity Disorder*', which many people struggling with sexual behaviours could relate to:

> an extreme and often life-long effort to conceal aspects of ones sexuality and the fear of revealing or having your authentic sexuality discovered, shamed, judged or punished by others. The primary symptoms of Sexual Authenticity Disorder are intense fear of discovery, sexual secrecy, dishonesty, and an attendant shame and guilt (2015, p. 118).

The more we view human sexual behaviour struggles through the wide aperture of pluralistic psychosexual psychotherapy, rather than the single lens of addiction, the more refined our formulation and the more effective our treatment approach will be.

In my spare time, I love reading and learning about cosmology. It gives me a sense of awe. I particularly admire the scientists working in that field because they sometimes have to put all their knowledge or assumptions back on the drawing board when they make a new discovery that questions the previous knowledge. I absolutely love the consistent curiosity, the passionate exploration, and the humility of open self-questioning. This is why I love science. I dislike a devout ideology because it is the opposite. People who are devout can literally make anything fit their beliefs and tune out what disagrees with their ideology. I think it is sad. But each to their own. I uphold my love for science by committing myself to re-writing this book entirely if there is a new scientific discovery that changes the nature of my understanding of compulsive sexual behaviours. I welcome that day if it comes. Since I will sadly never be an astronaut, I try to do my bit for science in my own little way.

References

American Association of Sexuality Educators, Counselors and Therapists (AASECT). Statement on Sex Addiction [Available Online]: https://www.aasect. org/position-sex-addiction.

Bering, J. (2013). *Perv: the sexual deviant in all of us*. London, UK: Penguin Random House.

Berlin, H.A. and Hollander, E. (July 2008). Understanding the differences between impulsivity and compulsivity. *Psychiatric Times*, 25(8), 58–61.

Braun-Harvey, D. and Vigorito, A.M. (2016). *Treating out of control sexual behavior: rethinking sex addiction*. New York: Springer Publishing Company.

Carnes, P. (1983) and (2001). *Out of the shadows: understanding sexual addiction*. Center City, Minnesota: Hazelden.

Cooper, M. and McLeod, J. (2011). *Pluralistic counselling and psychotherapy.* London: Sage Publications.

Donaghue, C. (2015). *Sex outside the lines.* Dallas, TX: BenBella Books.

DSM-5. *Diagnostic and statistical manual of mental disorders.* 5th ed. Arlington, VA: American Psychiatric Association.

Foa et al. (1980). Differential effects of exposure and response prevention in obsessive-compulsive washers. *Journal of Consulting and Clinical Psychology,* 48(1), 71–79.

Fous, G. (2015). *Decoding your kink.* Galen Fous, MTP, ISBN10: 1518659535, ISBN13: 978-1518659539.

Hall, P. (2019). *Understanding and treating sex and pornography addiction.* Abingdon, Oxon: Routledge.

Hartmann, M. (2020). The totalizing meritocracy of heterosex: subjectivity in NoFap. *Sexualities (June 2020).* Sage. https://doi.org/10.1177/1363460720932387.

ICD-11. International Classification of Disease. 11th revision. *World Health Organisation.* [Available Online]: https://icd.who.int/en.

ICD-11. International Classification of Disease. 11th revision. *World Health Organisation.* Link to the statement on CSBD by The Medical Services Advisory Committee. [Available Online]: https://icd.who.int/dev11/proposals/l-m/en#/http://id.who.int/icd/entity/1630268048?readOnly=true&action=DeleteEntityProposal&stableProposalGroupId=854a2091–9461-43ad-b909–1321458192c0.

Lewis, M. (2015). *The biology of desire.* New York, NY: Public Affairs.

Ley, D. (2012). *The myth of sex addiction.* Lanham, Maryland: Rowman & Littlefield Publishers.

Lindsay et al. (1997). Controlled trial of exposure and response prevention in obsessive-compulsive disorder. *British Journal of Psychiatry,* 171(Aug 1997), 135–139.

Magnanti, B. (2012). *The sex myth: why everything we're told is wrong.* London: Phoenix.

Maté, G. (2018). *In the realm of hungry ghosts: close encounters with addiction.* London, UK: Penguin Random House.

Prause et al. (2017). Data do not support sex as addictive. *The Lancet. Correspondence,* 4 [Available Online]: www.thelancet.com/psychiatry (Accessed: December 2017).

Sex Addicts Anonymous. (2005). International Service Organization of SAA. 3rd ed.

Chapter 2

The diagnosis of compulsive sexual behaviour disorder

In the first chapter, I discussed that the disorder framework is not entirely helpful but I think it is important that we understand what the current ICD-11 diagnostic criteria for the Compulsive Sexual Behaviour Disorder (CSBD) are. A close read of the CSBD diagnostic criteria reveals that most clients won't meet all of the conditions for the disorder, inversely offering us a tool to de-pathologise our clients. Most clients presenting with sexual behaviours that feel out of their control will be more accurately described as having Compulsive Sexual Behaviours, (CSB), rather than 'Compulsive Sexual Behaviour Disorder' (CSBD), if, indeed, we need to label them at all. The ICD-11 diagnosis criteria are:

> Compulsive sexual behaviour disorder is characterized by a persistent pattern of failure to control intense, repetitive sexual impulses or urges resulting in repetitive sexual behaviour. Symptoms may include repetitive sexual activities becoming a central focus of the person's life to the point of neglecting health and personal care or other interests, activities and responsibilities; numerous unsuccessful efforts to significantly reduce repetitive sexual behaviour; and continued repetitive sexual behaviour despite adverse consequences or deriving little or no satisfaction from it. The pattern of failure to control intense, sexual impulses or urges and resulting repetitive sexual behaviour is manifested over an extended period of time (e.g. 6 months or more), and causes marked distress or significant impairment in personal, family, social, educational, occupational, or other important areas of functioning. Distress that is entirely related to moral judgments and disapproval about sexual impulses, urges, or behaviours is not sufficient to meet this requirement.

Why is it so hard to meet the disorder criteria?

1   The disorder doesn't apply for intense urges and impulses that do not result in repetitive unwanted sexual behaviours, nor behaviours that are not as a direct result of uncontrolled sexual urges and impulses. Although

most clients do report strong urges and unwanted sexual behaviours, they are usually able to control their behaviours if the intense urge happens at a time when sex is not socially possible (otherwise, we would be seeing people having sex all over the place, all the time).

2 Most clients reporting CSB have perfectly good functioning life skills even if they are often preoccupied by their sexual thoughts or behaviours. If a client enjoys a lot of sex, they are usually very good at maintaining their personal hygiene.

3 Many people do not attempt to reduce their repetitive sexual behaviours until after they are caught by their partner. If there was no risk of getting caught many would happily continue their sexual behaviours, indicating that they derive enough satisfaction from it. They may think '*I shouldn't be doing this*' but they do it anyway because the motivation to meet their sexual needs trumps the motivation to keep to their agreed relationship boundaries with their partner. If this is the case, it is not a disorder, it is an erotic conflict. Most people do not engage in sexual behaviours that do not produce any satisfaction or any pleasure. We can observe the same phenomenon in the context of binge eating. Some people may binge on biscuits because they like the taste and therefore derive pleasure from it. You will probably never meet a binge eater compulsively eating a slab of butter, because it doesn't taste good.

4 A majority of clients come to therapy after they get caught by their partner. There is a question over inability to control those urges resulting in repetitive sexual behaviours or choosing not to control the behaviours because they produce pleasure. It is usually the latter.

5 If people can have repetitive sexual behaviours over an extended period of six months or more and not get caught, it usually means they are highly functioning and very much in control; it takes much planning and organisation to hide sexual behaviours from a partner. Clients report marked distress and significant impairment in personal areas of their life when they face a separation after they got caught, not before, which also rules out the diagnosis for the disorder.

6 It is not possible to diagnose the disorder if the client feels sexual shame, moral judgement or disapproval from a partner, society, families, religious groups, and so on. For example, a client may repetitively visit a Dominatrix sex worker because he derives much pleasure from BDSM practices. When his partner discovers the behaviour they tell him they are disgusted by it. The client then feels great distress at his behaviour and wants to stop. This client cannot be diagnosed with the disorder. Similarly, if a client thinks they are 'porn addicts' after reading an anti-porn book, they wouldn't meet the disorder either.

Grubbs et al. (2020a) support the moral judgment and disapproval as an exclusion for the disorder by demonstrating that moral incongruence positively predicts self-reported compulsivity in pornography use. The study shows that:

> moral incongruence was a substantive and robust predictor of self-reported compulsivity. These results underscore the contention that personal morality may influence individuals' self-perceptions of their sexual behaviours which, in turn, may complicate efforts to accurately diagnose compulsive sexual behaviour disorder.

In summary, the population who would meet the full current ICD-11 diagnostic for the disorder is rare. Although many people will come to therapy with a self-diagnosis of 'sex addiction' after completing some online tests, now that we have a diagnostic guide, we, psychotherapists, can reassure clients that most of them won't have a pathology, without dismissing their struggles. Psychotherapists will do best by their clients in formulating CSB as symptoms of underlying issues for which there is a wide range of psychosexual and psychotherapeutic treatment, rather than a disorder in itself.

As a diligent clinician, I take it as my duty to use the appropriate clinically endorsed term to give the correct information to clients so that they can make an informed choice about their psychological and sexual health care. Ley upholds the same clinical excellence:

> Language is important. If we don't believe that something is an addiction, then let's not call it an addiction. To adopt a term we disagree with, simply because it is popular or sells books, brings significant baggage. When doctors, therapists and other educated, trained and titled experts use words in a professional manner, we give those words credibility. While the public might use concepts in nonspecific ways, applying them as metaphors, in the mouths of doctors, they become diagnoses, labels, sentences, and condemnations (2012, p. 20).

Using the correct term means using the correct treatment. Every fire may look the same but they are not the same. Some need a water-based extinguisher, others need a powder-based one, depending on the nature of the fire. Using the wrong extinguisher can actually make the fire worse. This is the same principles with sexual compulsivity. Symptoms may look like an addiction, but it is not, according to the available science. The sexual behaviour that is problematic has to be evaluated by clients themselves. A client may say that their repetitive visits to sex workers is a problem but their pornography use is not. We, clinicians, are not to tell clients what is problematic or not.

The affective system and the deliberative system

Braun-Harvey and Vigorito (2016) use Haidt's metaphor of the elephant and its rider to describe two distinct brain systems: the affective system and the deliberative system. The affective system (elephant) runs automatically without conscious decisions. It is linked to our autonomic nervous system which regulates bodily functions, including sexual arousal. It is activated by our survival instinct and motivated by meeting our primal needs. Braun-Harvey and Vigorito explain that the affective system

> includes our sense of wanting, our desire to acquire something or to engage in an action (2016, p. 60).

On the other hand, our deliberative system (rider) is the one that makes conscious decisions and intellectually evaluates situations. As the affective system is linked to our survival instinct, it trumps the deliberative system; the rider is much smaller than the elephant. The rider and the elephant have to be in a relationship together in order to function properly. It is the role of the rider to build the trust with the elephant. It is an ongoing daily relationship. With this metaphor, we can better understand the relationship that we have with our erotic self. If the rider is made of sexual shame, sexual oppression and unhelpful morality, they will beat up the elephant, which can then rebel and become irresponsive to the rider.

Once people learn how to ride their elephant, the next step is to know where they both want to go. As clients get to know their Erotic Template well, they might discover that they have an interest in kink, for example. But if the path in which they are currently riding is vanilla monogamy it can potentially mean that their journey will be rocky because they may not be on the track that suits them. This struggle is what Braun-Harvey and Vigorito describe as the "*erotic conflict*". We all have erotic conflicts to varying degrees because we all have conflicts with our wanting and needing. A similar phenomenon is observed in the eating disorder field. The more one deprives themselves of food they like and enjoy, the more they set themselves up for a binge. The pleasure hunger is as important as the nutritional hunger. If the pleasure hunger isn't met, it eventually rebels against the deprivation and once the binge starts people describe feeling out of control. This is why the success rate of people going on diets is low. The same process happens with thoughts. The more we force ourselves to stop thinking about a behaviour, the more this behaviour is likely to increase. Interestingly, a study by Johnston et al. (1999) found that people who supress thoughts about chocolate are more likely to have chocolate.

Freud (1962) identified what he called the Id, Ego and Super Ego. In Freud's terms of the 'pleasure principle' the Id is where the instinctive components of our personality live, including our erotic impulses. The Ego is the decision-making part of our mind that is adapted by the external world. It is the voice of reason. The Super-Ego is the moralistic and prohibitive voice, often learnt from parents, which attempts to control the Id, especially the parts that our society finds uncomfortable, such as sex. We, therapists, must pay attention not to unconsciously have clients internalise us in their Super Ego. It is, however, important to engage with the Ego part of the client helping them listen to their Id and their Super-Ego so that they can make sense of their erotic conflicts for themselves. In the area of sexuality and compulsive sexual behaviours the Super-Ego will be supercharged with moralistic views and shame which will inform clients' sense of being 'out of control'.

Whether there is the presence of a sexual compulsivity problem or not, we are creatures of contradictions. It is our human nature. We want to eat the cake and we want to stay thin. We want the security of monogamy and we want the excitement of a flirt with a stranger. We want to have more time for sleep and we want to be on social media until 1am. Take a moment to think of your own contradictions.

The language of abundance

Many clients with CSB will already have a deprivation script constructed from childhood. Encouraging clients to avoid sexual stimuli and become erotically avoidant reinforces a deprivation script. Such strategies implicitly suggest that clients should not be exposed to their erotic conflicts. It isn't realistic. Living a good life is acquiring the skills to manage stress, anxiety, and adversities. Having a good sex life is learning the skills to manage erotic conflicts. We don't learn anything by avoiding things. This is basic psychotherapy knowledge. Suzanne Iasenza (2020) writes about helping clients deconstruct sex with *"the sexual menu"* where people can define different items of sensuality, sexuality and eroticism. They can choose to engage with some items of the menu or not at any particular time. I like this idea very much as it promotes the language of abundance. With this method, there is no avoidance and no deprivation. Clients can enjoy their banquet.

Predisposing, precipitating and maintaining factors of sexual compulsivity

Lew-Starowicz et al. (2019) suggests that emotional dysregulation is a core predisposing factor of CSB. Winters et al. (2009) concurs that men who were generally good at regulating their emotions were more able to regulate their sexual arousal. They also found that the precipitating and maintaining factors of CSB may not be the heightened sexual arousal per se but the distress that they feel in managing those intense feelings. Clients with good emotional regulation skills may not feel as distressed by intense sexual thoughts, feelings and needs whereas people with less emotional regulation could be more distressed at managing them. A study by Carvalho et al. (2015) supports the idea that problematic sexual behaviours is associated with a perceived lack of control over sexuality and moralistic attitudes rather than high levels of sexual desire and activity. A constant worry about sexual desire, arousal and behaviours may be the chronic unpleasant emotions that require the need for the repetitive pleasure-focused behaviour which maintains compulsivity. The theory of metacognition (Wells, 2009) is useful in this context in understanding that worry and rumination produce psychological and emotional disturbance.

The clients' ongoing dismissal of their Erotic Template and the mis-management of their erotic conflicts are often the components that maintain sexual compulsivity. Helping our clients accept and respect their Erotic Template is a key element to psychological well-being. There are other factors that can predispose, precipitate and maintain sexual compulsivity such as unresolved trauma, unresolved psychosexual problems, attachment disruption, poor self-esteem, narcissistic traits and high sexual desire. These will be examined in Part 2 of this book.

Sex as mood enhancer

There is a popular narrative that sex for the purpose of lifting moods is '*wrong*'. It is another incorrect message that members of the public often absorb. People will then think something is wrong with them if they feel sexual to improve their moods. To be clear, there is nothing wrong with having sex, partnered or solo, to lift moods. Orgasms in themselves have mood lifting properties. Isn't it great? Why not use it plentifully? One of the maintaining factors of sexual compulsivity, as we will explore, is to use sex as a way to regulate emotions. It is easy to misinterpret it as '*people should not have sex to lift their moods*'. It is not so. The problem is when sex is the *only* way that people have to regulate their emotions. Part of the treatment is to help clients add tools to regulate emotions alongside having sex rather than stopping anything.

Beyond the frontiers of 'sex addiction'

It is anxiety-provoking indeed to go against the grain and challenge the well-established 'sex addiction' experts. Whilst the 'sex addiction' clinics multiply, whilst the pornography panic grows, the science doesn't follow. Grubbs et al. (2020b) examined the body of research on 'sex addiction' over the past 25 years in a ground-breaking extensive review which further questions the validity of the 'sex addiction' conceptualisation:

much of this work is characterized by simplistic methodological designs, a lack of theoretical integration, and an absence of quality measurement.

Now that we are in a new decade, I invite clinicians to make a choice:

1   Do you want to be unquestioning of 'experts' and be a devout follower of a concept that ignores available science in order to stay with your comfortable view of sexuality or
2   Do you want to be a clinician led by the available science and challenge your knowledge for the purpose of continuous advancement and striving to offer better treatments to clients, even if the science goes against your personal beliefs?

I believe my 'sex addiction' colleagues are well-meaning therapists working hard to help their clients. We all work towards the same goal. My ambition is not to change therapists' minds, but simply to offer my colleagues some food for thoughts and a space to reflect. I invite my colleagues to keep being curious about sexology and to keep learning. Nissen-Lie et al. (2015) proposes that a self-doubting therapist is a better therapist!

References

Braun-Harvey, D. and Vigorito, A.M. (2016). *Treating out of control sexual behavior: rethinking sex addiction*. New York, NY: Springer Publishing Company.

Carvalho et al. (April 2015). Hypersexuality and high sexual desire: exploring the structure of problematic sexuality. *Journal of Sexual Medicine*, 12(6), 1356–1367. https://doi.org/10.1111/jsm.12865.

Freud, S. (1962). *The ego and the id*. New York: W.W. Norton & Company, ISBN-10: 0393001423.

Grubbs, J.B., Kraus, S.W., Perry, S.L., Lewczuk, K., and Gola, M. (2020a). Moral incongruence and compulsive sexual behaviour: Results from cross-sectional interactions and parallel growth curve analyses. *Journal of Abnormal Psychology*, 129(3), 266–278. https://doi.org/10.1037/abn0000501.

Grubbs et al. (2020b). Sexual addiction 25 years on: A systematic and methodological review of empirical literature and an agenda for future research. *Clinical Psychology Review*, 82, 101925, Elsevier. https://doi.org/10.1016/j.cpr.2020.101925.

Haidt, J. (2006). *The happiness hypothesis: finding modern truth in ancient wisdom*. New York, NY. Basic Books.

Iasenza, S. (2020). *Transforming sexual narratives: a relational approach to sex therapy*. New York, NY, Abingdon, Oxon: Routledge.

ICD-11. International Classification of Disease. 11th revision. *World Health Organisation*. [Available Online]: https://icd.who.int/en.

Johnston et al. (1999). Supressing thoughts about chocolate. *International Journal of Eating Disorders*, 26(1).

Lew-Starowicz et al. (2019). Compulsive sexual behaviour and dysregulation of emotion. *Journal of Sexual Medicine Review*, PMID: 31813820, doi: 10.1016/j. sxmr.2019.10.003.

Ley, D. (2012). *The myth of sex addiction*. Lanham, Maryland: Rowman & Littlefield Publishers.

Nissen-Lie et al. (2015). Love yourself as a person, doubt yourself as a therapist? *Clinical Psychology & Psychotherapy*, 24(1).

Wells, A. (2009). *Metacognitive therapy for anxiety and depression*. New York, NY: The Guilford Press.

Winters, J., Christoff, K., and Gorzalka, B.B. (2009). Conscious regulation of sexual arousal in men. *Journal of Sex Research*, 46(4), 330–343. doi: 10.1080/00224490 902754103.

Chapter 3

The science of sexology

I would like to enumerate a few points here that I learnt from sexology and psychotherapy. By no means do these points summarise the entirety of the available psychosexual knowledge. But I thought it was important to start here to introduce you to the general direction of my thinking in sexual compulsivity.

1   Sexual behaviours are not addictive. There is not enough evidence to support the concept of addiction.
2   Sexual compulsivity has more comorbidity with impulsive, compulsive and mood disorders but not with behavioural or substance addictions as shown by Fuss et al. (2019), which supports the International Classification of Disease (ICD-11) diagnostic criteria for Compulsive Sexual Behaviour Disorder (CSBD).
3   It is widely accepted in sexology that there is no normative standard for sexual activity even if it appears uncommon, as Bering reminds us in his delightful book *Perv: the sexual deviant is all of us* (2013). Castellini et al. (2018) assert that paraphilic thoughts and behaviours are not considered sexual deviancy, but need to be viewed from a broad spectrum of human sexuality to understand what may be problematic for clients.
4   Sexual compulsivity seeks to resolve unmet needs, either emotionally, relationally or sexually. It also attempts to resolve attachment problems. It is maintained in a complex system of various psychological and physiological processes (Barcenas, 2017; Spenhoff et al., 2013).
5   The problematic sexual behaviours are symptoms of underlying disturbances. If we are behaviour-focused, we won't treat the problem. The unwanted sexual behaviours are a coping strategy. It is important not to encourage clients to give them up before new ones are established. Human beings try to achieve homeostasis, thus their unwanted sexual compulsivity is maintained for a very good reason, as indicated by Gestalt theories (Clarkson, 2004).
6   Compulsive sexual behaviour problems can be treated with permanent change using a humanistic and pluralistic modality combining classic

psychotherapy and sexology. A thorough understanding of the client's erotic mind is crucial, which means that the treatment needs to be psychosexually oriented (Morin, 1995).

7   Sexual fantasies are not dangerous, no matter how extreme they may be. They can be an invaluable window into discovering our erotic world. People do not always want to act on their sexual fantasies (Lehmiller, 2018). Having sexual fantasies is a common strategy to bring ourselves to sexual arousal or to escape from something difficult. There is no pathology with either of these mechanisms. Fantasies are not necessarily a gateway to unwanted sexual behaviours. Asking clients to stop having sexual fantasies about unwanted behaviours is inefficient and can in fact increase the desire for those unwanted sexual behaviours.

The Erotic Template and the Painter's Palette

The Erotic Template is all the elements of someone's erotic mind that is functional, sexually pleasurable, wellbeing enhancing, erotically potent and fulfilling. I believe it is important that we first help clients understand it before we find out what is a problem for them and what makes their sexual behaviour compulsive. All the elements that are in the client's Erotic Template are not to be tampered with. In Part 2 of this book, I will explain how to assess a client's Erotic Template.

When I deliver clinical trainings on sexuality, I often start the day asking delegates: *'what is your favourite dessert?'*. The answers are usually specific: *'warm brownie with vanilla ice cream on the side'*. *'Sticky toffee pudding with just a little bit of custard'*. *'Lemon tart from the special French bakery'*. *'My mother's apple pie'*. People's Erotic Template is similar. It is unique and specific. I use the imagery of a painter's palette. Some people will have a few dominant colours on their palette. For some, one of the dominant colours might be Kink, for others it might be Vanilla. Next to these dominant colours, there will be all sorts of other colours too, less dominant, some only a tiny dot. Inviting clients to explore their palette and find out about their colourful Erotic Template is a very good start of therapy because without that knowledge, we cannot assess what is problematic. When clients have a better understanding of their Erotic Template, they can already start to make some meaning of it. As we will see later, sexual compulsivity doesn't survive in meaning. With this approach, we can already start to treat clients' sexual compulsivity even before discussing the problems.

Some of the colours on clients' palette are dominant and permanent. These are the ones closely related to their sexual orientation. Some other colours move from being dominant to less dominant, depending on a person's sexual and relational development, age, different priorities and values, different experiences and so on. The painter's palette changes as we change through life. Keeping in touch and staying curious with our palette and our Erotic Template requires erotic intelligence, which clients can learn in therapy.

The four cornerstones of eroticism

In his pioneering book *The Erotic Mind* (1995) Jack Morin gifts us with the concept of the "*four cornerstones of eroticism*" to help us guide our clients in understanding their erotic world. My interpretation of these are:

1   **Longing and anticipation**. Some find delayed gratification erotically potent. Looking forward to something with sexual and romantic anticipation can awaken the erotic. Similarly, being apart from your partner for a period of time may bring up longing, which can also revitalise sexual and romantic desire and arousal.
2   **Violating prohibition**. We are socialised to follow rules for the good reason that it is what makes a society function. But, often, our erotic is interested in what is politically incorrect, or to indulge in something that you would not want anyone to know about. Violating prohibition can be a fertile ground for vibrant erotic. For some, it may be having an affair. For others it could be having sex outdoors, or an activity such as dogging. In social situations, men and women may want to be perceived and thriving as equal. However, in the bedroom, there may be sexual potency in breaching this social etiquette by consensually 'using' one person for the pleasure of the other. Heterosexual men engaging in sexual contact with other men, rape fantasy, describing yourself as a 'cumdump', the list goes on. The transgressive is erotic.
3   **Searching for power**. We don't have to identify as kinky or be a member of the BDSM community to play with power in the bedroom. A doggy style position when one consensually pushes the face of the other into the pillow can be considered as power play and strongly erotic for people. Other power play may take the form of role plays such as doctor and patient, boss and employee, and so on.
4   **Overcoming ambivalence**. Some people experience the push and pull between partners as erotic. Ambivalence may be described as being with the unknown, which can create a low-level anxiety. The release of that anxiety can produce sexual arousal. The 'hard-to-get' type of play may be both within power play and overcoming ambivalence. Cuckolding, a sexual practice in which one experiences sexual arousal from their partner having sex with someone else (Lehmiller, 2018) may belong to this cornerstone too. Gay men can find bareback sex extremely arousing because of the uncertainty of the HIV transmission, the erotic that they can get away with it is potent.

The ten types of erotic boosters

Throughout the years of my work I have identified what I call the ten types of erotic boosters. Whilst the four cornerstones of eroticism can make up the main colours of a client's palette, the boosters are what makes those colours brighter or they can be an entry point that activates the Erotic Template.

1 **Visual.** Some people are more visual than others. Their primary entry to sexual arousal may be through what they see. It could be seeing a person with a particular type of clothes or shoes. It may be the lighting in a room. Some people like to see tattoos, or make-up or a particular type of hair colour. Some enjoy looking at genitals they find beautiful.
2 **Olfactory.** Some people are more sensitive to scents. It can be scent of candles or flowers. For some people it is the scent of sweat or other bodily odour.
3 **Auditory.** Some people can experience an erotic boost with sounds. It may be the sound of club music, or the sound of heavy breathing or a partner moaning with pleasure. For some, it can be the sound of dirty talking.
4 **Touch.** Some people get sexually aroused primarily through touch. It may be skin to skin touch, or it could be touching through a specific material like silk, velvet or leather. Some people get aroused with the sensation of their bodies wearing a particular fabric. The primary arousal of touch also includes sexual stimulation. Some people become aroused only when they stimulate erogenous zones.
5 **Stress.** It may be counter-erotic for many, but in fact stress can be a powerfully arousing for some people. The experience of stress can awaken the erotic as a demand to process the stress through sexual activities or pleasure.
6 **Boredom.** This is also not usually discussed in terms of sexual arousal. As human beings, we try to avoid boredom, so it can be an erotic booster as a means to fill up the time.
7 **Emotional.** Some people are more likely to have an erotic boost when they feel certain emotions. For some people, it may be feeling safe and secure. For others it may be the opposite, being in a risky or edgy situation. For some people, it is the feeling of love. For others it is the intoxicating feeling of infatuation. Sometimes, it can actually be the feeling of anger that awakens the erotic.
8 **Hormonal.** Hormones can affect our experience of arousal. Men may feel more sexual in the morning because there is a testosterone spike then. Women may feel more sexual at certain times of the month depending on their hormonal cycle. The hormonal make up of a person may produce spontaneous sexual desire.
9 **Fantasy.** Some people are fantasy-based, which means story-based. Many people enjoy an erotic boost with role plays, or just by imagining

a story or a particular event. It can be fictional fantasy; imagining something that could never happen in real life (in 2019, the second top search on PornHub was 'Alien'). Or it could be the fantasy of a memory, a sexual activity that clients did in the past.

10 **Environment.** Some people need the place to be right for their erotic boost. Usually, there are many places that will do for sex, but some people can have some peak turn-ons with particular places such as outdoors. For others it may be in the kitchen, in the bathroom, in the office, in a public toilet or in a sex club.

These ten types of erotic boosters are non-pathological and part of the diversity of human existence. Some therapists might incorrectly think that a client being aroused through visual is wrong as they might assume it is objectification; or they might think it is problematic to be aroused by boredom or fantasies. Keeping the erotic boosters in mind can help clients understand their erotic processes and normalise some of their sexual urges. Someone who is genuinely self-aware of their Erotic Template and erotic boosters can make conscious choices to engage in sexual activities, either solo or with partners.

The somatic erotic pathways

In my work, I have identified that people respond to what I call somatic erotic pathways. They are the entry points of sexual desire and arousals that emerge from past pleasurable experiences. Memories are powerful, we remember them with our mind, with all of our senses and with our bodies. Some pleasurable memories will embed in us in what I call erotic somatic markers. When clients encounter such marker, they will instantly and automatically feel sexual. Ben had fond memories of being held by his mother when she chewed a eucalyptus gum. The smell of eucalyptus automatically sends an urge to be touched in that moment. Patrick has a memory of a fantastic sexual experience on a sunny day in a nudist beach once. When he feels the similar sunny temperature, he has a sexual urge. Fiona had one of her best orgasmic experiences with a man who had piercing blue eyes, looking at her as he brought her to orgasms. Now, she feels a sexual urge when she sees men with the same eye colour. These somatic erotic pathways are not pathological. It is just the way that our brain works with memories. The psychological problem occurs when clients feel shame about eroticism that emerge instantly.

The six principles of sexual health

When clients have a better understanding of their Erotic Template, we can guide them to think about what might be outside of it that is problematic for them. The six principles of sexual health is a good guide to understand what is functional first, before thinking about what is not. Clients can assess their own sexual behaviours thinking about whether they fit within the six principles. The rationale behind this is that if we are behaviour-focused, we can easily insert our own sexual morality. However, if we are principle-focused, it is easier to think about sexual behaviours non-judgmentally. It also helps to reduce sexual shame.

Braun-Harvey and Vigorito (2016) conceptualise compulsive sexual behaviours as *"Out of Control Sexual Behaviours"* (OCSB). Their treatment plan is a sexual health model. They describe extensively the six principles of sexual health and how they weave it in their clinical practice in their pioneering book *Treating Out Of Control Sexual Behavior, Rethinking Sex Addiction*. I will offer here my own interpretation of the principles:

1   **Consent.** It is the explicit permission to have sexual contacts with other people. Consent can be withdrawn at any time. Betty Martin offers the model of the Wheel of Consent on her website (bettymartin.org). Martin teaches us that consent is not only saying 'yes' or 'no' to touch, it is having clarity of the details of what we are consenting to. Martin explains that we can consent to gift our body for someone's pleasure, or we can touch for our own pleasure. All the people involved in the sexual activity have to be clear about what they're doing and what they're consenting to, at all times. As soon as there is a doubt or a discomfort, the participants can request to pause and re-establish clarity or they can choose to withdraw consent altogether, which must be respected immediately.

2   **Nonexploitation.** Exploitation is using our power to coerce others. It can be an emotional, psychological and sexual manipulation. Sometimes, exploiting people can resort to strategies such as gaslighting. Infidelity can be seen as exploitation of the relationship because the betrayed person does not have all the information to make choices about what they consent to in the relationship.

3   **Protection from HIV, STIs and unwanted pregnancy.** This may seem simple, yet it is not. In the UK, we have the best contraception technology yet there is a high rate of unwanted pregnancy. Avoiding unwanted pregnancy requires an active willingness to learn accurate sex education and plan properly. Some women have serious side effects from contraceptive pills but there are other solutions too. Protection from HIV is changing. In the gay community the advancement of pre-exposure prophylaxis (PrEP) means that many gay men can protect themselves against HIV without using a condom, however it doesn't protect them against other STIs. For people living with HIV, adhering to their medications brings their viral load to be undetectable and they cannot transmit the virus to others. This is fantastic progress in sexual health.

4 **Honesty.** This principle starts with oneself. Being honest with ourselves can be a hard task that therapy can help with. Honesty includes knowing our Erotic Template even if some of the colours on the palette don't fit with society's norms. We have to be honest with our relational self too. Some of us have a relational need that does not fit monogamy. We have to approach honesty with ourselves with compassion; getting to know ourselves in depth non-judgmentally is a gift to ourselves, even if it is sometimes hard to face. Once we are honest with ourselves, we can be honest with others. Being candid is a great gift of love to our partner(s), even when it is hard to do. It takes great courage from clients to reveal to a 'vanilla' partner that they are turned on by kink, for example (not to say that vanilla is not a gorgeous and complex flavour). There is a great risk that the partner may be repulsed which brings a fear of rejection for clients. But on the other hand, it offers opportunities for the partner to get to know them better.

5 **Shared values.** This is a principle that encourages honest conversations with partner(s). We all have values and they are usually precious to us. It is important for clients to have a dialogue with their partner(s) about their specific values, including specific sexual activities, how to initiate sex, the components of morality, religion, gender-biased thinking, and so on. Partner(s) deciding to engage in sexual and relational encounters must make sure they share those wonderful intimate moments with others of the same values. Failure to do so can bring great wounding. For example, if someone has Christian values that pornography is unacceptable, it is best to have that conversation explicitly before they make a relationship commitment rather than assuming that the partner has the same values because they met in Church. If a client has a consensual non-monogamy need, they must make sure they find someone with the same need and values, otherwise they can feel 'trapped' in monogamy and blame their partner for it when it was they who might not have been clear in the first place.

6 **Mutual pleasure.** Sexual pleasure is one of the most dismissed and unspoken components of sexual health. Donaghue (2015) writes about our society being largely sex-negative and sends prolific pleasure-negative messages. Isn't it strange, given that it is the most common motivator for having sex? Sex education tends to focus on avoiding diseases and reproduction, but it is not all there is about sexual health. Thankfully, we have wonderful sex-positive public figures in the UK such as award-winning broadcaster Alix Fox (@alixfox). Mutual pleasure does not mean having orgasms at the same time. In fact, trying to orgasm at the same time can bring more anxiety than pleasure. People can have orgasms at different times and still meet the mutual pleasure principle. Pleasure does not necessarily mean orgasm. Pleasure is about being fully present in the moment, with touch, skin-to-skin

pleasure, fun, laughter, exploration, fingers, tongues, role plays and so on. Pleasure doesn't need to be penetration-focused, and it doesn't even require an erection. For some, pleasure can be cybersex pleasure, a practice that became more popular since the COVID-19 pandemic. Meeting this principle does involve the activities being pleasurable for all involved. If at any point someone feels that something is not quite right in the chosen activity, then the honesty and consent principle has to kick in. Discussing mutual pleasure can be intimate and hot, definitely sexier than enduring something that doesn't feel right.

Braun-Harvey and Vigorito remind us of the WHO definition of sexual health (2006):

> Sexual Health is the possibility of having pleasurable and safe sexual experiences, free of coercion, discrimination and violence.

Clinicians can have powerful conversations with their clients about what their breach of sexual health principles means to them, thereby guiding them towards good sexual health. I think it more useful to discuss a client's sex life with the sexual health lens rather than the medicalised binary of what is 'healthy' or 'unhealthy' where we may fall into polarised views that are potentially unnecessarily pathologising.

The erotic equation

The erotic equation is another gift from Morin (1995). He teaches us that our erotic mind may be governed by the following equation:

> Attraction + Obstacle = Excitement

Esther Perel (2017) agrees:

> the risk of being caught doing something naughty or dirty, the breaking of taboos, the pushing of boundaries – all of these are titillating experiences (…) we are most intensely excited when we are a little off-balance, uncertain (2017, p. 161).

This phenomenon is not only observed in the erotic world, it is prevalent in other situations that is themed with our desire and hunger, thus it could also be named the equation of desire. I'm sure we can all relate to really wanting dessert when it is the least accessible. In the peak of COVID-19 times, when the country started its lockdown and shops quickly ran out of supply, we suddenly became quite excited about that juicy tomato that was left on the shelf, or indeed, toilet paper.

Morin's equation can inform how psychotherapists can work with clients presenting with sexual compulsivity. If therapists make the goal to stop unwanted sexual behaviours, encourage clients to avoid 'triggers' and not think of sexual fantasies, the therapy may become the obstacle that will make that very unwanted sexual behaviour more exciting and harder to resist. The negative impact of this is that clients can feel more hopeless and broken for not being able to stop their behaviours, thinking they're failing therapy, when in fact, it may be the therapy that fails them.

The Coolidge effect

The Coolidge effect is a popular term taken from a joke (probably fictional) about the US President Mr and Mrs Coolidge being taken to a chicken farm separately. Mrs Coolidge noticed how the rooster was vigorously sexually active and asked the farm guide to make sure that Mr Coolidge took note of this behaviour. When the guide talked to Mr Coolidge about it, he said to the guide to make sure his wife took note that the rooster was sexually active with different hens. The Coolidge effect is the phenomenon of having renewed sexual energy when a new person is sexually available even if the usual partner is still sexually available. It is thought to be a biological evolutionary phenomenon that increases the chances of reproduction with new partners. The Coolidge effect has been observed with animals (Wilson et al., 1963) and with humans (O'Donohue and Geer, 1985). Interestingly, a study showed that sperm is of better quality when exposed to novelty, which confirms the evolutionary theory (Joseph et al., 2015). The Coolidge effect is not only a male sexual behaviour, women like novelty too (Kelley and Musialowski, 1986).

People can sometimes misinterpret their experience of the Coolidge effect for a sign of sexual compulsivity, especially when it is observed from the point of view of the long-term partner. For example, men can often be scolded for looking at other women in the street. I am not talking about intimidating women by staring and wolf whistling at them. This is different. I'm talking about a fleeting moment of erotic tantalisation at noticing someone new and attractive. If there has been a past infidelity or a history of compulsive sexual behaviours, the Coolidge effect might be perceived as dangerous, unwanted and the 'gateway' to more compulsivity. It is not always the case. In fact, the more one is prescribed not to look at attractive people, the more that person will become attractive and enticing (Morin's erotic equation).

The Coolidge effect can also explain why pornography is so popular. If you want novelty, porn can certainly deliver! People in a long-term relationship might actually benefit from watching pornography together if they are both into it.

In the context of a relationship being hurt by sexual compulsivity, as in any other committed relationships, it is more useful to help clients accept and manage the Coolidge effect rather than ignoring or criticising it.

The philosophy of sex-positivity and pleasure-positivity

Many clinicians say that they are sex-positive but I wonder how many have examined what it really means. The International Society for Sexual Medicine (ISSM) offer a description of sex-positivity on their website:

> having positive attitudes about sex and feeling comfortable with one's own sexual identity and with the sexual behaviours of others.

My definition of sex-positivity is:

1 Exploring, Embracing and Celebrating the Erotic Template (sexual fantasies, thoughts, desires, arousals and behaviours) without judgement.
2 Accepting that one person's erotic turn-on can be another person's erotic turn-off.
3 Being loyal to sexual authenticity: being aware of your erotic palette, and to keep in touch with it as it changes over time, with new experiences and maturing.
4 Understanding sexual boundaries. What is legal and consensual. What feels good and what doesn't feel good.
5 Understanding that sex is not addictive.
6 Understanding, accepting and celebrating the wide range of gender, sexuality and relationship diversity, including transgender people, asexuality, bisexuality, queer, kinks, fetishes, polyamory, etc.
7 Being willing to learn more about gender, sexuality and relationship diversity when you think you have a blind spot.
8 Understanding sexual behaviours need to align with the person's core values and sexual integrity.
9 Accepting and celebrating all body shapes.
10 Being willing to challenge sex-negativity and to promote sex-positivity and pleasure-positivity with our peers and communities.

Therapists can have their own definition of what sex-positivity means to them. It is also important to understand what sex-positivity is not. It is not when we judge other people's sexual behaviours based on our own ideas about it. These definitions of sex-positivity are essential to work efficiently with compulsive sexual behaviours as a philosophy to commit oneself to.

In addition to being sex-positive, therapists working with sexual compulsivity need to be pleasure-positive. The World Association for Sexual health (WAS) made a declaration on sexual pleasure (2019):

> Sexual pleasure should be exercised within the context of sexual rights, particularly the rights to equality and non-discrimination, autonomy and bodily integrity, the right to the highest attainable standard of health and freedom of expression.

In my consulting room, I find that I have to support my clients with their birth right of freedom of sexual expression and their sexual pleasure. It is mostly relevant for clients who belong to a minority group such as LGBTQ+ population and the Black, Asian and Minority Ethnic (BAME) community.

Chris Donaghue makes a very good point about our society's biases and how we have morals on the hierarchy of pleasurable activities:

> One can watch football or sitcoms on television all day, but to watch erotica (or what many call "porn") regularly is considered addictive behavior. Many will use a film or a book to "check out" for relaxing self-care but are shamed if they do the same with masturbation. Travel for sightseeing is great, but to travel for sexual variety isn't supported (2015, pp. 12–3).

Sexual orientation, fetish and kink

In the spirit of sex-positivity, we need to stay open to the possibility that for some people, their Erotic Template may have a dominant colour of kink or fetish. Some people may experience their fetish and kink as a sexual activity they enjoy whilst others may identify it as a sexual orientation.

Kort offers a definition of sexual orientation:

> The innate, main focus of one's sexuality, often with the understanding that a sexual "orientation" is also affectionate, spiritual, emotional, relational, and psychological. It is enduring, lasting, and unchanging (2018, pp. 398–9).

Moser (2016) asserts that there are "significant psychological consequences if the sexual attraction and arousal is denied or repressed or if it is explored and fulfilled."

Sprott and Williams (2019) find that Bondage/Discipline, Dominance/ Submission, Sadism/Masochism (BDSM) practices share similar character-istics to the definition of sexual orientation and argue that for some people it may be perceived as such whilst for some others, it may be a "*serious leisure activity*". The authors describe kink and fetish:

> Aspects of kink include eroticizing intense sensations (including but not limited to "pain"), eroticizing power dynamics and power differentials, enduring fascination with specific sensory stimuli including specific body parts or inanimate objects ("fetish"), role play or dramatizing erotic scenarios, and erotic activities that include heightened or altered states of consciousness.

Unfortunately, there are still many therapists who believe that people can be 'addicted' to BDSM because of past trauma. This is inaccurate and sex-negative. Shahbaz and Chirinos (2017) debunk common BDSM myths including:

> There is no research that indicates clients with BDSM have a greater history of past abuse or trauma that predisposes them to this form of sexual expression. The practice of BDSM itself does not cause distress and dysfunction in individuals (2017, p. 30).

BDSM is founded on the thorough understanding of consent and thus is one of the most conscious sexual practices. Nobody understands sexual boundaries and consent more than BDSMers! We, therapists, must differentiate between trauma-re-enactment and BDSM, these are different things. The conscious and deliberate resolution of trauma via BDSM practices is not essentially pathological, although Langdridge and Barker (2007) caution that the "healing narratives" can be unhelpful too:

> For example, people may read such narratives as indicating that all BDSMers have been abused or traumatised in some way, that BDSM is a means to an ends for those who are psychologically damaged and that, as such, it can be discarded once some spurious goal of sanity has been reached (2007, p. 211).

The Shahbaz-Chirinos Healthy BDSM Checklist (2017) is an essential guide for therapists.

> Its primary aim is to explore (1) whether clients are engaging in BDSM consensually; (2) to assist clients in obtaining clarity about their reason, vision and philosophy of the practice of BDSM; and (3) the degree to which their values align with their practices (2017, Appendix A).

There is much misunderstanding of kink in our psychotherapy profession; the BDSMers are particularly vulnerable to accidental conversion therapy (I discuss this in Chapter 5). It is paramount to be properly kink-aware in this work.

Reference

Barcenas, I. (2017). Literature review: attachment style and hypersexual disorder. *Journal of Sexual Medicine*, 14(5 Suppl 4), e280. https://doi.org/10.1016/j.jsxm.2017.04.351.

Bering, J. (2013). *Perv: the sexual deviant in all of us*. London, UK: Penguin Random House.

Braun-Harvey, D. and Vigorito, A.M. (2016). *Treating out of control sexual behavior: rethinking sex addiction.* New York: Springer Publishing Company.

Castellini et al. (2018). Deviance or normalcy? The relationship among paraphilic thoughts and behaviors, hypersexuality, and psychopathology in a sample of university students. *Journal of Sexual Medicine,* 15(9), 1322–35. https://doi.org/10.1016/j.jsxm.2018.07.015.

Clarkson, P. (2004). *Gestalt counselling in action.* 3rd ed., London: Sage Publications.

Donaghue, C. (2015). *Sex outside the lines.* Dallas: BenBella Books.

Fox, A. (2020). [Available Online]: Instagram: @alixfox.

Fuss et al. (2019). Compulsive sexual behaviour disorder in obsessive-compulsive disorder: prevalence and associated comorbidity. *Journal of Behavioral Addictions,* 8(2), 242–8. Published online 2019 May 13. doi: 10.1556/2006.8.2019.23.

ICD-11. International Classification of Disease. 11th revision. *World Health Organisation.* [Available Online]: https://icd.who.int/en.

ISSM. What does "sex positive" mean? *International Society for Sexual Medicine.* [Available Online]: https://www.issm.info/sexual-health-qa/what-does-sex-positive-mean/.

Joseph, P. N., Sharma, R. K., Agarwal, A. et al. (2015). Men ejaculate larger volumes of semen, more motile sperm, and more quickly when exposed to images of novel women. *Evolutionary Psychological Science,* 1, 195–200. https://doi.org/10.1007/s40806-015-0022-8.

Kelley, K. and Musialowski, D. (1986). Repeated exposure to sexually explicit stimuli: Novelty, sex, and sexual attitudes. *Archives of Sexual Behavior,* 15, 487–98.

Kort, J. (2018). *LGBTQ clients in therapy: clinical issues and treatment strategies.* New York: W.W. Norton & Company.

Langdridge, D. and Barker, M. (2007). *Safe, sane and consensual.* Basingstoke, Hampshire: Palgrave Macmillan.

Lehmiller et al. (2018). The psychology of gay men's cuckolding fantasies. *Archives of Sexual Behavior,* 47(2018), 999–1013.

Lehmiller, J. (2018). *Tell me what you want.* London: Robinson.

Martin, B. (2019). Wheel of consent. [Available Online]: https://bettymartin.org.

Morin, J. (1995). *The erotic mind.* New York: HarperCollins Publishers.

Moser, C. (2016). Defining sexual orientation. *Archives of Sexual Behaviours,* 45, 505–8. The Official Publication of the International Academy of Sex Research. doi:10.1007/s10508-015-0625-y.

O'Donohue, W. T. and Geer, J. H. (1985). The habituation of sexual arousal. *Archives of Sexual Behavior,* 14, 233–46.

Perel, E. (2017). *The state of affairs: rethinking infidelity.* London: Yellow Kite.

Porn Hub insights. (2019) year in review. [Available Online]: https://www.pornhub.com/insights/2019-year-in-review.

Shahbaz, C. and Chirinos, P. (2017). *Becoming a kink aware therapist.* New York, NY, Abingdon, Oxon: Routledge, Taylor & Francis.

Spenhoff et al.. (2013). Hypersexual behavior in an online sample of males: associations with personal distress and functional impairment. *Journal of Sexual Medicine,* 10(12), 2996–3005. doi:10.1111/jsm.12160. Epub 2013 Apr 11.

Sprott, R.A. and Williams, D.J. (2019). Is BDSM a sexual orientation or serious leisure? *Current Sexual Health Reports*,11(2), doi: 10.1007/s11930-019-00195-x.

Wilson, J. R., Kuehn, R. E., and Beach, F. A. (1963). Modification in the sexual behavior of male rats produced by changing the stimulus female. *Journal of Comparative and Physiological Psychology*, 56, 636.

World Association for Sexual Health (WAS). Declaration of sexual pleasure. [Available Online]: https://worldsexualhealth.net/declaration-on-sexual-pleasure/.

Chapter 4

Compulsive watching of pornography and masturbating

The fear and the research

There is so much confusion about pornography at the moment. There seems to be a cultural and social panic about it. Much of what is online and in books on the subject demonises porn, creating fear. The instant access to pornography through devices is relatively recent. It is easy to be in panic about it if we don't understand it, we think it is everywhere, only a few taps away, invading the private space of our homes.

People are free to think of pornography whichever way they want to think of it, watch it or not watch it. It doesn't bother me. I'm neither pro-porn nor anti-porn. However, what bothers me is the vast amount of 'fake news' about porn that is unscientific, grossly misleading the public. I'd like to bring some clarity to the debate.

It is common to point the finger at porn for relationship and sexual problems that clients present with. Unfortunately, focusing on helping clients to stop watching pornography might not fix people's sexual issues, their relationship problems or their sense of well-being. Most importantly, focusing on stopping watching pornography won't teach clients anything about themselves, their erotic mind, or how to achieve psychological and psychosexual wellbeing. It won't teach clients anything about what is really going on in their intimate relationships.

Many people talk about pornography, but what do we mean by it? Surprisingly, it seems that it is complex to find a good definition of it. McKee et al. (2020) arrive at two 'incompatible' themes in the definitions, and suggest that we should use the definition that fits best with what we want to use it for:

> (1) Sexually explicit materials intended to arouse, and (2) Pornography is not a thing but a concept, a category of texts managed by institutions led by powerful groups in society in order to control the circulation of knowledge and culture, changing according to geographical location and period.

Rea (2001) defines pornography as 'communicative materials (picture, paragraph, phone call, performance, etc.)', explaining that the person accessing pornography wants to be sexually aroused by that content. The second component to Rea's definition is that pornography is used or treated as such 'by most of the audience for which it was produced'.

The similarities in the attempts to define pornography are:

1 Pornography is a wide range of materials including images, texts and conversations, with the primary aim of sexual arousal.
2 It is a cultural perception that identifies what pornography is by most of the audience of that culture.

The complexity of defining pornography has reminded me of the book 'SEX' by Madonna, which was perceived by many as pornography then, but probably would not be now. In some other cultures, a sexy poem may be considered pornography, whereas in the UK we tend to think of pornography as hardcore and explicit sexual films. It makes sense that the definition changes over time as cultural norms change.

Let's de-bunk some popular myths about pornography. I would like to stress again that these are not my personal opinions, there are my clinical opinions based on scientific research.

Pornography does not make a bad society

Data shows that sexual crimes are lower in areas where there is greater access to porn (Ley, 2016, p. 36). This phenomenon is observed widely. In 2019, the gay press reported many priests and preachers against homosexuality getting caught on gay hook-up apps soliciting sex with other men. This is a case of projective identification (Klein, 1998). Promoting homophobia is an attempt to force others to repress their sexuality for the purpose of disowning the parts of their sexuality that they perceive as undesirable. The easy access to pornography offers our society a window through which adults can satisfy their curiosity and explore their sexuality. It is a good window into which one can get to know one's erotic world. Most people watch the pornography that they find titillating, even if it is a small part of their Erotic Template. People don't tend to keep watching something that repulses them. Ley explains:

If someone watches porn showing something they find distasteful, it has no impact on their behavior or desires.

Nelson and Rothman (2020) assert:

pornography itself is not a crisis. The movement to declare pornography a public health crisis is rooted in an ideology that is antithetical to many core values of public health promotion and is a political stunt, not reflective of best available evidence.

A fascinating study by Kutchinsky (1991) demonstrates that there was no increase in the number of rapes perpetrated in West Germany during the time when pornography was made legal and became widely available. More recently, Burton et al. (2010) found that there was no correlation in juvenile sexual abusers and their exposure to pornography regarding the age at which the abusers started abusing. Similarly, a study by Dawson et al. (2019) found no corroboration between male adolescents' pornography use and sexual aggressiveness. Mellor and Duff (2019) concur that there is no evidence of a relationship between pornography and sexual offenses. In fact, they found that men who offend report less exposure to pornography. Equally, pornography viewing does not increase the harm perpetrated to the victim.

Pornography does not create objectification

Objectification is making a person an object of sexual desire and gratification. Ley writes:

> Objectification is a human process that we use in our interactions with others. It is neither good nor bad; it just is (2012, p. 86).

Lehmiller (2018) published his research on sexual fantasies indicating that both men and women naturally objectify in order to connect to their erotic world and their fantasies. According to Lehmiller's survey, heterosexual women want their fantasy man to be taller than average with an athletic body but not too muscle bound, brown or black hair and more well-endowed than average (2018, pp. 132–3). Women who objectify are not considered a threat in our society. I am sure we can all remember the popular Diet Coke advert in which women objectify a handsome man taking his t-shirt off. That kind of objectification is totally acceptable. Objectification can help with sexual desire and sexual arousal. Moreover, Lehmiller shares a fascinating component of the outcome of his research: men and women fantasise more about their current romantic partners than famous people, including porn stars:

> There's a very good reason why our partners in the real world are our most common partners in fantasy, and it's because our fantasies often include a strong emotional component. The vast majority of men and women rarely fantasise about emotionless sex (2018, p. 143).

This adds an extra dimension to our understanding of sexual fantasies and porn watching. When people watch pornography, they are not only wanting to watch an explicit sexual act, they also want to imagine what they feel if they were doing that act themselves, therefore it is an emotional process too. McKee (2005) conducted a study in Australia and showed that women are not objectified in a way that it denies their human agency in mainstream pornographic videos.

Pornography does not cause relationship problems

Gillath et al. (2008) found the opposite phenomenon:

> exposure to sexual stimulus motivates people to initiate and maintain close relationships.

It seems that erotic honesty fosters a greater ability to have positive conflict resolution. The Gottman Institute teaches us on their website the four behaviours that are most corrosive to relationships which they call *The four horsemen of the apocalypse*: (1) criticism, (2) defensiveness, (3) contempt and (4) stonewalling. In the context of watching pornography, I would add sexual shaming, high moralistic views, power struggles, low self-esteem, distorted beliefs about sex and relationships and insecurities as the main culprits to relationship problems. In other words, it is not the pornography that destroys relationships but how people think about it based on how it activates their insecurities and moralities.

Staley and Prause (2013) found that watching erotic films increased people's desire to be close to their current partner. This concurs with Lehmiller's research results mentioned earlier (2018). Grov et al. (2011) found that couples watching adult websites together experienced enhanced sexual arousal, openness to try new things and were associated with positive consequences. Maddox et al. (2011) reached a similar conclusion in their study that couples watching pornography together reported more dedication and sexual satisfaction than those watching pornography alone. Balzarini et al. (2017) did not find any evidence that exposure to attractive images affected men's view of the partner's sexual attractiveness or their love for them. Bennett et al. (2019) published a study confirming that:

> pornography consumption was not significantly associated with sexual desire for one's partner. Such finding is important, as it reinforces recent research that shows that pornography has minimal effects in modern romantic relationships (...) though feelings of guilt regarding pornography use negatively predicted sexual desire.

The study conducted by Maas et al. (2018) also shows that men who are more accepting of pornography report higher relationship satisfaction. Gaber et al. (2019) found that watching pornography was good for people's sex lives with reports of '*coital likelihood is higher on viewing days*' with reports of higher sex drive for their partner. According to all these studies, we can easily conclude that shaming men for watching pornography may be what creates relationship problems rather than pornography itself. Moreover, Perry and Longest (2019) found that there was no difference in entering marriage amongst those who watch pornography frequently and those who did not, further disproving the moral panic that porn somehow causes chaos in relationships. A recent research by Liu et al. (2020) showed that perceived risks and perceived infidelity were negatively related to engagement in online sexual activity.

Pornography does not induce erectile dysfunction

This is a popular view that is fiercely inaccurate yet instilling so much fear, especially in young male adults who have anxiety about their erections. Erectile dysfunction is a common presentation in men. Hackett et al. (2018) report a large European study found the prevalence of erectile dysfunction to be 19% in men aged 30–80 years; whilst other studies found the presentation ranging from 22% in the United States to 10% in Spain. The psychological factor is usually anxiety-related if there isn't an underlying medical problem. Putting fear of porn in these men is likely to increase their anxiety! I often hear clients who experience erection problems say that pornography is the easiest way they can enjoy their sexuality without the anxiety of performance. It may therefore appear to be more enjoyable than partnered sex. Rather than blaming pornography for erectile dysfunction, we might do a better service to our clients to have conversations about what else is going on for them and offer them a more suitable psychosexual therapeutic service. If it is not performance anxiety, could it be their partner's disapproval of them watching pornography that brings the erection difficulties? The vast body of scientific research on this subject is clear: there is no evidence that pornography causes erectile dysfunction or any other sexual dysfunction (Prause and Pfaus, 2015; Sutton et al., 2015; Klein et al., 2015; Landripet and Štulhofer, 2015; Grubbs and Gola, 2019; Berger et al., 2019).

Janssen et al. (2020) find that men who identify as 'hypersexuals' have no stronger responses to sexual stimuli than those who do not. There was also no evidence of negative mood on sexual arousal. This research replicates a growing body of research which finds no association between pornography watching and erectile functions. However, Cranney (2015) finds that pornography use had an impact on men's body image of penis-size dissatisfaction. Interestingly, the same study found no links between porn use and women's breast-size satisfaction.

Pornography does not lead to sexual violence towards women

Rasmussen and Kohut (2019) reported that people watching pornography had more egalitarian attitudes than those who did not. The difference in attitude was stronger with people who observed religious practices regularly. This population has a greater likelihood to experience moral incongruence when watching pornography. The study shows that this pattern was consistent across three egalitarian attitudes that was examined: attitude towards women in power, women in the workplace and abortion. Barak et al. (1999) conducted the first controlled study which found no relationship between substantial exposure to pornography and men's attitude towards women. Kohut et al. (2016) affirms that pornography users have more egalitarian attitudes towards women in position of power, or women's equal rights including abortion than those not watching pornography, interestingly. Jackson et al. (2019) published a study on the attitude of *"Porn superfans"* and found that they were no more sexist or misogynistic than the general population. Moreover, they had

> more progressive gender-role attitudes than the general public (...) Our results call into question some of the claims that porn consumption fosters de facto negative and hostile attitudes towards women.

A UK study published by Attwood and Smith (2010) in the *Journal of Law and Society* assert:

> Rather than address the particular structural factors and material realities which contribute to women's risk of violent attack and men's propensities to violence, the current political and legal climate seeks to demonize sexually explicit media for these crimes.

Of course, there is no denying that there is a dark side to pornography when it is made by people who traffic women, just as much as there is a dark side to the food industry putting poison in our food for financial profits. Yet, most of us consume processed food. Violent pornography can be a problem with people who already have views or desires that are sexually violent towards women. For those people, watching violent pornography may reinforce their pre-existing views. But not all pornography is bad. Most of the porn available isn't dark. Ley (2016) offers some helpful suggestions to navigate this. With a little bit of background check of porn companies, people can be safe in knowing they can watch ethical porn from legitimate production companies treating their performers with respect and paying them fairly. Pornography is adult entertainment. We don't need to watch it. I have spoken informally to many sex workers and adult film performers, many of whom report feeling empowered by their profession.

Pornography is not addictive

This is also a very popular belief. 'Pornography addiction' is being consistently rejected from all medical and psychological bodies as there is a lack of clinical evidence of its existence. However, the psychological state of those watching porn is what needs to be considered, primarily their attitudes towards it, their sexual shame and their religious values. Kohut et al. (2017) assert that '*no negative effects*' was the highest research finding regarding the impact of pornography use. Perry (2019) cautions us that studies that do not take into account the role of masturbation are not properly sound studies on pornography. I think it is important to remind ourselves of this to quieten so much stentorian panic around the subject. The statistics of pornography use for 2019 offered by PornHub reveal that the average length that people spend watching pornography in one sitting is 10 minutes, which suggests that pornography is mostly used for masturbation. A recent study by Charig et al. (2020) finds that exposure to online pornography has no impact on any psychosocial factors including sexual functioning and mental well-being. Binnie and Reavy (2020) concur in their study concluding that pornography is not harmful. However, they suggest more research is done to develop a model that can help those struggling with pornography.

Dopamine is often mentioned as a way to make those anti-porn '*studies*' credible. The truth is that dopamine goes up when the brain notices something is novel (Schultz, 1992). Dopamine is actually great and healthy, but not special, it only means the brain is responding appropriately to novelty, which is a common feature of online porn. Leonhardt et al. (2020) find that pornography use is congruent with people's sexual desire. On the other hand, perceived compulsivity was associated with *obsessive and inhibited sexual passion*, which means that there is either an underlying mental health problem or shame about their sexual desire.

What is the problem with pornography?

If pornography is not the problem in itself, then what is the real problem? It is important to recognise that many people do struggle with their compulsive watching of pornography. It is easy for people watching pornography to stumble across something that had never been in the periphery of their thinking with only a click. If they happen to feel curious and a little tantalised by it, they might watch it for a few minutes longer than if they had no interests in it at all, in which case they wouldn't even spend a second watching it. It means that pornography can be a good tool for people to get to know their erotic mind in a lot more detail.

Whether we like it or not, young people are curious about sex. We cannot change that, no matter how uncomfortable it makes us feel. Watching pornography is adult entertainment and not appropriate for underage people. But there is a major lack of sex education. Parents feel awkward talking about sex. Children don't want to have sex education delivered by their own parents anyway. Teachers are equally uncomfortable talking about it. So where does it leave young people with a mind full of curiosity and questions about sex? Of course, they turn to pornography. It is definitely the wrong place for sex education. The inappropriate lessons they get from porn are: *'my penis should be big and hard all the time'*, *'vulvas should be hairless'*, *'men and women's body should look perfect'*, *'sexual intercourse should last for 30 minutes at least'*, and so on. All of these messages are so bad that they will set young people up for a lot of sexual and relationship problems. It is not a pornography problem, it is a sex education problem. We need more, inclusive sex education that is not part of the biology lesson on reproduction. There needs to be a course in itself about sexual pleasure, including same-sex relationships. It needs to be done by a qualified and experienced sex educator rather than a teacher who was unlucky enough to draw the short straw to get the hour of sex education ticked off the curriculum. Let's look at it another way: shall we say that fast food causes obesity and kills people? Shall we then ban all fast food and only have salad shops? Or is the problem due to people not knowing enough about nutrition, not knowing how to use fast food appropriately, not knowing how to cook? What if there was more food education and what if we taught every child how to cook properly? I think it would be more useful than demonising fast food. The same goes with pornography. I'm so pleased that the UK has now made inclusive sex education compulsory despite the protest of religious groups. It is a great step forward in protecting our children from harm. Gegenfurtner and Gebhardt (2017) provide evidence that the benefits of sex education which includes LGBTQ+ relationship and sexuality will be *overwhelmingly positive*.

It is important to remind ourselves that sexual rights are human rights. Sex education delivered at school is not about exposing children to sexual material too early but teaching some very important aspects of human rights and should be done as early as primary school age with teachings on consent and accepting diversity, through to high school with sexual health and sexual pleasure.

Compulsive watching of pornography is not about pornography. It is about underlying issues. Here are some of the most common ones:

Insecure relationship dynamics

Many women fear porn because of their insecurities; they can't compete with the porn actress: *'if my husband watches a blond actress and I'm brunette, it means he doesn't find me sexually attractive'*. As mentioned earlier, Lehmiller (2018) finds that people fantasise mostly about their partner and much less about porn performers. For some, porn is a way to imagine themselves having great sex with their partner. For others, it is a private world that is well boundaried and doesn't have an impact on their sexual feelings towards their partner. There is a similar phenomenon with men being threatened by women using sex toys fearing that the toy is a replacement of their penis because it can provide more pleasure than the penis; *'how can my penis compete with toy vibrations going for hours!'* Yet, most women enjoy their partner's penis and their sex toys in boundaried ways, without any dark motives of replacing their partner's penis. One of the sexual health principles is shared values. If clients have different values about porn and they are important to them, they may need to consider finding someone with the same values. Let's take another example: some people will only be in a relationship with someone who shares their political values, or they dietary values, or their status values. The same goes with the porn values.

Psychosexual issues

Most often, because of a lack of sex education and anxiety-filled first sexual experiences, erectile dysfunction, premature ejaculation or delayed ejaculation can be a struggle for many men. Most often, these psychosexual problems are what we call 'situational', they only occur in the situation where they are with a partner, not when alone. This is obvious as there is no need for anxiety of performance when alone. Porn does not create such dysfunctions. The dysfunctions come first and make porn a lot more pleasurable than partnered sex. Resolving these psychosexual issues involves fostering an anxiety-free sexual space and full acceptance with the couple, which can be almost impossible to achieve if one partner is very hurt by the use of porn, disapproving and angry.

Sexual shame

It is now well documented that the biggest struggle that people face with porn isn't actually the watching it or masturbating to it, but the shame they feel about it. Shame is a strong emotion that can propel some people to try to find a 'cure' for their porn problems. For some people, it is the guilt about masturbation that causes distress such as depression and erectile problems rather than pornography itself (Chakrabarti et al., 2002). In my consulting room, I see on a regular basis sexual shame dissolving as soon as I normalise masturbation behaviours and present them with the real science behind pornography. However, if a client's religious beliefs are really important to them, we have to respect it and help the client face their dilemma: either they make peace with their beliefs and porn or they can think about stopping watching porn to match their beliefs, with full awareness of why they ask themselves to stop: not because porn is bad, but because it doesn't suit their beliefs, much like a vegan would not eat bacon out of their important values rather than bacon being dangerous. In such case, it is also important to discuss with clients how they will meet their sexual curiosity and desires. Clinical psychologist Cameron Staley in his TEDx Talk (2019) makes the astute observation that our behaviours match what we believe about ourselves. He proposes that if people believe they are 'porn addicts' they are more likely to behave as such. The very label of 'porn addict' may be maintaining factor for some.

Volk et al. (2019) suggests that people who morally disapprove of their pornography use are more likely to label themselves as 'addicted' with a greater sense of depression and sexual shame. Moreover, the study finds that, as well as blaming pornography for their problem, these people are more likely to externalise their transgression onto others.

For a lot of people their problem with porn is value-based. You might love bacon but you also hate the way that pigs are slaughtered. If your animal rights value is stronger than your love for bacon, you can easily stop eating it. But if the animal rights value isn't that strong, you will struggle to stop eating bacon.

Self-soothing

For some people, watching porn and masturbation is a good way to soothe some emotions of stress, sadness, anger, boredom, for example. If it is the only method for soothing, porn watching and masturbation can feel compulsive. Individuals need to learn other ways to self-soothe so that they can have different strategies to deal with emotions, not just one. Porn watching and masturbation can then be one out of several methods of soothing and it will feel more in control.

Digisexuality

I believe that when clients access therapy because of their struggle with pornography, we can no longer ignore the emerging new sexuality called digisexuality as part of the client's clinical picture. Digisexuality is defined as:

> sexual experience that depends on the use of an advanced technology (McArthur and Twist, 2017).

The *First Wave Digisexuality* uses mediating technology which means that they use technology for a new or enhanced sexual activity with a human partner. *First Wave digisexuality* includes online pornography, social media, online dating, hook-up apps, and webcamming. I can imagine these behaviours have become even more popular since the COVID-19 pandemic. The

Second Wave Digisexuality uses immersive technology which means that the sexual activity does not rely on human partners. These include robots or virtual reality. The *Second Wave Digisexuality* is currently quite rare, predominantly because of the cost of technology required. As technology improves, we may see more people who self-identify as 'digisexuals', that is to say people

> whose preferred form of sexual experiences and relating is via immersive technologies and which need not involve a human partner (McArthur and Twist, 2017).

Twist and McArthur (2020) defined digital health as:

> having pleasurable and safe technology-based experiences, free of coercion, discrimination, and violence. For digihealth to be attained and maintained, the rights of persons online and offline must be respected.

Similar to the six principles of sexual health, Twist and McArthur (2020) identified five principles of digihealth:

1   Consent
2   Protection from exploitation and harm
3   Honesty
4   Privacy
5   Pleasure

Using the digihealth core principles, we can help clients identify what their struggles are, and it can give us a guide on how we can address it. Similar to the six principles of sexual health, when we look at these we are less likely to insert moral judgements. However, it does require the therapist not to be a technophobe and to believe that a functional attachment to technology can be part of well-being.

Reference

Attwood, F. and Smith, C. (2010). Extreme concern: regulating 'dangerous pictures' in the United Kingdom. *Journal of Law and Society*, 37(1), 171–88.

Balzarini et al. (2017). Does exposure to erotica reduce attraction and love for romantic partners in men? Independent replications of Kenrick, Gutierre and Goldberg (1989) study 2. *Journal of Experimental Social Psychology*, 70, 191–7.

Barak et al. (1999). Sex, guys, and cyberspace: effects of internet pornography and individual differences on men's attitudes towards women. *Journal of Psychology & Human Sexuality*, 11(1), 63–91.

Barnett, J. (2016). *Porn panic! sex and censorship in the UK*. Alresford, Hants.: Zero Books.

Bennett et al. (2019). The desire of porn and partner? Investigating the role of scripts in affectionate communication, sexual desire, and pornography consumption and guilt in young adults' romantic relationships. *Western Journal of Communication*, 83(5), 1–21.

Berger et al. (2019). Survey of sexual function and pornography. *Military Medicine*.

Binnie, J. and Reavy, P. (2020). Development and implications of pornography use: a narrative review. *Sexual and Relationship Therapy*, 35(2), 178–94.

Burton et al. (2010). Comparison by crime type of juvenile delinquents on pornography exposure: the absence of relationships between exposure to pornography and sexual offense charasteristics 1. *Journal of Forensic Nursing*, 6(3), 121–9.

Chakrabarti et al. (2002). Masturbatory guilt leading to severe depression and erectile dysfunction. *Journal of Sex & Marital Therapy*, 28, 285–7.

Charig et al. (2020). A lack of association between online pornography exposure, sexual functioning, and mental well-being. *Sexual and Relationship Therapy*, 35(2), 258–81.

Cranney, S. (2015). Internet pornography use and sexual body image in a Dutch sample. *International Journal of Sexual Health*, 27(3), 316–23.

Dawson et al. (2019). Adolescent sexual aggressiveness and pornography use: a longitudinal assessment. *Aggressive Behavior*, 45(6), 587–97.

Gaber et al. (2019). Effect of pornography on married couples. *Menoufia Medical Journal*, 32(3), 1025.

Gegenfurtner, A. and Gebhardt, M. (2017). Sexuality education including lesbian, gay, bisexual, and transgender (LGBT) issues in schools. *Educational Research Review*, 22, 215–22.

Gillath et al. (2008). When sex primes love: subliminal sexual priming motivates relationship goal pursuit. *Personality and Social Psychology Bulletin*, 34(8), 1057–69.

The Gottman Institute. *The four horsemen of the apocalypse*. [Available Online]: https://www.gottman.com/blog/the-four-horsemen-recognizing-criticism-contempt-defensiveness-and-stonewalling/.

Grov et al. (2011). Perceived consequences of casual online sexual activities on heterosexual relationships: a US online survey. *Archives of Sexual Behavior*, 40(2), 429–39.

Grubbs, J.B. and Gola, M. (2019). Is pornography use related to erectile functioning? Results from cross-sectional and latent growth curve analyses. *The Journal of Sexual Medicine*, 16(1), 111–25.

Hackett et al. (2018). British Society for Sexual Medicine Guidelines on the Management of Erectile Dysfunction in Men – 2017. *International Society for Sexual Medicine: The Journal of Sexual Medicine*, 15(4), 430–57.

Jackson et al. (2019). EXPOsing men's gender role attitudes as porn superfans. *Sociological Forum*, 34(2).

Janssen et al. (2020). Sexual responsivity and the effects of negative mood on sexual arousal in hypersexual men who have sex with men (MSM). *The Journal of Sexual Medicine*.

Klein, M. (1998). *Love, guilt and reparation and other works 1921-1945*. Vintage.

Klein et al. (2015). Erectile dysfunction, boredom, and hypersexuality among coupled men from two European countries. *The Journal of Sexual Medicine*, 12(11), 2160–7.

Kohut et al. (2016). Is pornography really about "making hate to women"? Pornography users hold more gender egalitarian attitudes than nonusers in a representative American sample. *The Journal of Sexual Research*, 53(1), 1–11.

Kohut et al. (2017). Perceived effects of pornography on the couple relationship: initial findings of open-ended, participant-informed, "bottom-up" research. *Archives of Sexual Behavior*, 46(2), 585–602.

Kutchinsky, B. (1991). Pornography and rape: theory and practice? Evidence from crime data in four countries where pornography is easily available. *International Journal of Law and Psychiatry*, 14(1–2), 47–64.

Landripet, I. and Štulhofer, A. (2015). Is pornography use associated with sexual difficulties and dysfunctions among younger heterosexual men? *The Journal of Sexual Medicine*, 12(5), 1136–9.

Lehmiller, J. (2018). *Tell me what you want*. London: Robinson.

Leonhardt, N.D., Busby, D.M., Willoughby, B.J. (2020). Do you feel in control? Sexual desire, sexual passion expression, and associations with perceived compulsivity to pornography and pornography use frequency. *Sexuality Research and Social Policy*. https://doi.org/10.1007/s13178-020-00465-7.

Ley, D. (2012). *The myth of sex addiction*. Lanham, Maryland: Rowman & Littlefield Publishers.

Ley, D. (2016). *Ethical porn for dicks: a man's guide to responsible viewing pleasure*. Berkeley, CA: ThreeL Media.

Liu et al. (2020). Influence of online sexual activity (OSA) perceptions on OSA experiences among individuals in committed relationships: perceived risk and perceived infidelity. *Sexual and Relationship Therapy*, 35(2), 162–77.

Maas et al. (2018). A dyadic approach to pornography use and relationship satisfaction among heterosexual couples: the role of pornography acceptance and anxious attachment. *Journal of Sex Research*, 55(6), 772–82.

Maddox et al. (2011). Viewing sexually-explicit materials alone or together: association with relationship quality. *Archives of Sexual Behavior*, 40(2), 441–8.

McArthur, N. and Twist, M.L.C. (2017). The rise of digisexuality: therapeutic challenges and possibilities. *Sexual and Relationship Therapy*, 32(3/4), 334–44.

McKee, A. (2005). The objectification of women in mainstream pornographic videos in Australia. *Journal of Sex Research*, 42(4), 277–90.

McKee et al. (2020). An interdisciplinary definition of pornography: results from a Global Delphi Panel. *Archives of Sexual Behavior*, 49, 1085–91.

Mellor, E. and Duff, S. (2019). The use of pornography and the relationship between pornography exposure and sexual offending in males: a systematic review. *Aggression and Violent Behavior*, 26.

Nelson, K.M. and Rothman, E.F. (2020). Should public health professionals consider pornography a public health crisis? *American Journal of Public Health*, 110(2), 151–3.

Perry, S.L. and Longest, K.C. (2019). Does pornography use reduce marriage entry during early adulthood? Findings from a panel study of young Americans. *Sexuality & Culture*, 23(2), 394–414.

Perry, S.L. (2019). Is the Link Between Pornography Use and Relational Happiness Really More About Masturbation? Results From Two National Surveys. *Journal of Sex Research,* 57(1), 2020.

PornHub insights. (2019) year in review. [Available Online]: https://www.pornhub.com/insights/2019-year-in-review.

Prause, N. and Pfaus, J. (2015). Viewing sexual stimuli associated with greater sexual responsiveness, not erectile dysfunction. *The Journal of Sexual Medicine,* 3(2), 90–8.

Rasmussen, K.R. and Kohut, T. (2019). Does religious attendance moderate the connection between pornography consumption and attitudes towards women? *Journal of Sex Research,* 56(1), 38–49.

Rea, M.C. (2001). What is pornography? *NOÛS,* 35(1), 118–45.

Schultz, W. (1992). Activity of dopamine neurons in the behaving primate. *Seminars in Neuroscience,* 4(2).

Staley, C. and Prause, N. (2013). Erotica viewing effects on intimate relationships and self/partner evaluations. *Archives of Sexual Behavior,* 42(4), 615–24.

Staley, C. (2019). *TEDx Talks: changing the narrative around the addiction story.* [Available Online]: https://www.youtube.com/watch?v=mNGg5SMcyhI.

Sutton et al. (2015). Patient characteristics by type of hypersexuality referral: a quantitative chart review of 115 consecutive male cases. *Journal of Sex & Marital Therapy,* 41(6), 563–80.

Twist, M.L.C. and McArthur, N. (2020). Introduction to special issue on digihealth and sexual health. *Sexual and Relationship Therapy,* 35(2), 131–6.

Volk et al. (2019). The moderating role of the tendency to blame others in the development of perceived addiction, shame, and depression in pornography users. *Sexual Addiction & Compulsivity,* 26.

Chapter 5

Being ethical

First do no harm

We, clinicians, must take care not to confuse our clinical opinions, which should be evidence-based, and our personal opinions. Most people have strong opinions about sex and relationships. If one of your friends breaks up with their partner, notice how quick it is to form a personal opinion on their relationship and sex life. When your friend gets cheated on, notice how even quicker you place a judgement. Whilst ethics and morals are often used interchangeably, they have a different meaning. Ethics are rules provided by an external source such as our professional membership bodies. Morals are an individual's own principles of what is right and wrong. A therapist may morally disagree with watching pornography or visiting sex workers, but ethically they are not to judge the client for these behaviours and must honour their autonomy.

Let's take a moment for self-reflection and think about the following:

1   What is your personal judgment about going to sex clubs on a weekly basis?
2   What is your personal immediate reaction about barebacking?
3   What are your personal thoughts and feelings about anonymous sex?
4   What are your personal thoughts and feelings about visiting sex workers?
5   What are your personal thoughts about watching pornography daily?

In your own personal life, you are obviously free to have any thoughts and feelings you want. You can even be judgmental. But think about the impact of your personal thoughts on your enquiries and interventions when you are with clients who disclose some of the behaviours mentioned above. Do your enquiries and interventions belong to your personal opinion or do they belong to your professional ethical framework? If you assume that a sexual behaviour is a problem because it is something that you either morally disagree with or don't understand, how does it influence your enquiries?

1   If you think that going to a sex club on a weekly basis is bad, are you less likely to hear that it might not be a problem for the client? You might not hear that the client isn't coming for help for this particular sexual behaviour.
2   If you think that barebacking is dangerous or dirty, are you less likely to be curious about it and enquire about the pleasure of it?
3   If you are repulsed by anonymous sex, might you not think about exploring what the benefits of such behaviours are for the client?
4   If you hate the thought of visiting sex workers, might you not be willing to hear what the client positively gains from this behaviour?
5   If you morally disagree with watching pornography, might you automatically assume that the client's sexual and relational problems are caused by the pornography?

The basic principle of psychotherapy is to respect client's autonomy and not tell clients what to do with their lives. Psychotherapy is a place of introspection, inner understanding, and meaning making.

Therapists know that when we speak to a client we can send subconscious psychological messages to them. By focusing on stopping unwanted sexual behaviours as the primary goal, we send a psychological message: '*Your sexuality is wrong*'.

Our clients suffering with CSB are likely to have at least one subconscious story embedded in shame. Sending the psychological message to clients that their sexuality is wrong is likely to increase the shame story, and therefore cause harm.

Accidental 'conversion therapy'

Mike is turned on by kink, particularly being dominant having sex with submissive women. He thinks he's a 'sex addict' because his wife asks him to have non-kinky sex and he doesn't feel aroused so much. In his 12-step programme, kinky sex and male dominance over submissive women is wildly misunderstood; it is perceived as a component of 'the disease'. Mike is persuaded to believe his kinky side is 'abnormal', which will need to change. He feels shame each time he has a turn-on thought about kink, and he tries very hard to cut this off from himself. He also tries hard to feel aroused by vanilla sex, and feels that he is failing every time, reinforcing his beliefs of being diseased and gradually feeling hopeless about being 'a good man'. What does this story remind you of? Doesn't it sound like 'conversion therapy'?

'Conversion therapy' is based on the beliefs that heterosexuality is the only normal sexual expression and anything that doesn't follow it is therefore deviant. As such, in the 'conversion therapy' ideology, homosexuality is believed to be deviant, a disease and abnormal. The belief is that 'conversion therapy' can cure homosexuality. It is usually a 'therapy' offered within a religious context by a 'spiritual counsellor'. In the UK, all the major psychological bodies, including COSRT (College of Sexual and Relationship Therapists) agreed on a Memorandum of Understanding that 'conversion therapy', also known as 'gay cure' or 'reparative therapy', is not to be promoted or practiced as it is unethical and causes great harm. In May 2020, the United Nations of Human Rights published a report calling on the global ban of the practice (www.ohchr.org).

Is it possible that Mike, a heterosexual man, could be a victim of a variation of 'conversion therapy'? 12-step-oriented programmes may encourage a client who has a more diverse sexuality, such as kink, fetishes, consensual non-monogamy, and so on, to believe that these things are undesirable and should be changed, when in fact, they are absolutely normal, functional, and a part of a large natural sexuality diversity. For some people, their fetish and kink is a part of their Erotic Template that is closely related to their sexual orientation. I would like to invite psychotherapists to think further about preventing 'conversion therapy' as it might still be widely practice, not only with the LGBTQ+ population but also with the heterosexual population under the name of 'sex addiction'. I would like to be clear about one thing here: I don't believe that all therapists offering a 'sex addiction' treatment are unethical. But I think that it is possible that many well-meaning and excellent therapists can practice 'conversion therapy' accidentally, as described eloquently by Julie Sale in her blog post for The Contemporary Institute of Clinical Sexology (2019). Since Dr Joe Kort invited me on his popular podcast *Smart Sex Smart Love* on this subject in January 2020, numerous people living in the UK reached out to me to tell me about the psychological harm they suffered from their 'sex addiction' treatment and 12-step 'sex addiction' programmes. I fear that there are many more harmed clients who do not speak up.

I respect people's autonomy to choose the option of going to a SAA or SLAA meeting. I do not stop anybody from making their own choices. But clinicians need to think carefully about it and not make an automatic recommendation to access one of those meetings. We therapists need to be held accountable for our recommendations. It is our responsibility not to send clients to support groups where there is a high likelihood of sexual shame, sex-negativity, over-pathology and misinformation incongruent with psychotherapy and sexology.

The problem with one-size-fits-all programmes

Babette Rothschild cautions us:

> Treatment failures are particularly hidden when professionals – for whatever reason- are limited to adhering to a single model (...) In such circumstances, if something goes awry in the therapy, the blame must go

to the client. How could the method be blamed if it is the only one available? (2017, p. xix).

When clients don't respond to our clever and informed interventions, therapists often think their client is 'treatment resistant', 'difficult', 'in denial', and so on. Instead, I invite therapists to question themselves:

How am I not understanding the client?
What does the client need that I haven't offered yet?
What is my blind spot and my limitations?
Where is my knowledge gap?
What other modalities can I look into that might fit the client better?
Is my framework helpful?
Does my personal opinion get in the way of my professional one?

As psychotherapists, isn't it our job to find the right treatment for our clients? Or is it the clients' job to fit in our way of working? Ok, it was a tricky question. I believe it is a bit of both, actually. We can only offer clients what we are qualified to practice, and we have to be clear with clients how we can help them. But I also think it is our job as therapists to keep questioning ourselves, keep expanding our knowledge, keep learning about other modalities and keep sharpening our skills.

References

COSRT. Good Therapy. Code of Ethics and Practice. (2019). *College of Sexual and Relationship Therapists. (2019)* [Available Online]: cosrt.org.uk.

Kort, J. (2020). *Smart sex smart love podcast.* Helping clients recovery from the trauma of 'sex addiction' treatments. Interview with Silva Neves. [Available Online]: https://smartsexsmartlove.com/2020/01/13/silva-neves-on-helping-clients-recover-from-the-trauma/.

United Nations Human Rights (2020). Report on conversion therapy: independent expert on protection against violence and discrimination based on sexual orientation and gender identity. [Available Online]: https://www.ohchr.org/EN/Issues/SexualOrientationGender/Pages/ReportOnConversiontherapy.aspx.

Rothschild, B. (2017). *The body remembers, Volume 2. Revolutionizing trauma treatment.* New York: W.W. Norton & Company.

Sale, J. (2019). Are you an accidental conversion therapist? *Blog from The Contemporary Institute of Clinical Sexology.* [Available Online]: https://www.theinstituteofsexology.org/blog/are-you-an-accidental-conversion-therapist.

Part II

The pluralistic and sex-positive approach

Assessment of the diverse population

Chapter 6

Assessments

It is important to have a solid assessment and a unique clinical formulation of the client's difficulties if the clinician is to choose the appropriate treatment. The formulation of the client's clinical picture consists of:

1   **An initial assessment** to meet the client and discuss their current sexual behaviour problems. It is an opportunity for the psychotherapist to do an initial check if the client has indeed a sexual compulsivity problem or if it is something else, but without making a rushed formulation.
2   **A sexology assessment** to help clients identify their unique Erotic Template (chapter 3). This is the frame of clients' erotic picture, that is to say what therapists must not attempt to pathologise in order to remain in ethical practice. It is a shame reduction process. Within this assessment, we can identify if clients have unresolved psychosexual problems that may be part of the clinical picture.
3   **A psychological assessment** to help clients discuss any traumas, adverse experiences in their past and their sexual and relational history that could contribute to their present sexual behaviour problems.
4   **A formulation** of an appropriate and unique treatment plan based on the thorough assessments. Psychotherapists can then begin to formulate the predisposing precipitating and maintaining factors of the client' sexual compulsivity.

Through these assessments I take into consideration all aspects of a client's life; the biological, psychological, social, cultural, psychosexual, spiritual and financial aspects in line with the pluralistic philosophy. My assessment process is not formulaic or based on structured questionnaires. I prefer to gather the information I need through conversations. That way, clients get a sense of being seen, heard and we can start to build a therapeutic relationship from the very first meeting. Some of you will prefer to use formal assessment protocols or documents. Do what works best for you and your current approaches to assessment. We are pluralistic after all. Some of the forms that you might find useful are the Sexual Sensation Seeking and

Sexual Compulsivity Scale (Burri, 2016); and the Adverse Childhood Experiences (ACE) score.

The initial assessment

The simple formula to assess the sexual behaviours that clients present to us as unwanted and compulsive is to follow the ICD-11 criteria. These initial questions primarily serve the purpose of assessing whether clients do have a sexual compulsivity problem or not. These clients may indeed have problems with their sexual behaviours, but it may not necessarily be sexual compulsivity. In the initial assessment I ask some or all of these questions:

1 When you have a sexual impulse or urge, how intense do you feel them on a scale of 0 to 10, 0 being nothing at all and 10 the most intense you can possibly feel them?
2 Are there some particular sexual impulses or urges that are more intense than others? If so, what is your rating on the scale of 0–10?
3 When you feel those sexual impulses or urges, what happens next?
4 When you feel those sexual impulses or urges, do you find it difficult to control them?
5 When you feel those sexual impulses or urges, do you remember being able to control them sometimes (when the situation is inappropriate for meeting the sexual urges, for example)?
6 How often do you have those intense sexual impulses or urges?
7 When you feel your sexual impulses or urges, do you always act on them sexually?
8 Are your sexual behaviours always as a result of your intense sexual impulses or urges?
9 Would you consider your sexual behaviours repetitive?
10 How much can you control your repetitive sexual behaviours on a scale of 0–10?
11 When you engage in your repetitive sexual behaviours, do they become the central focus of your life to the point of neglecting other areas of your life?
12 When you engage in your repetitive sexual behaviours, do they become the central focus of your life to the point of neglecting your health?
13 When you engage in your repetitive sexual behaviours, do they become the central focus of your life to the point of neglecting your work?
14 When you engage in your repetitive sexual behaviours, do they become the central focus of your life to the point of neglecting your personal care?
15 When you engage in your repetitive sexual behaviours, do they become the central focus of your life to the point of neglecting other important activities in your life?

16   When you engage in your repetitive sexual behaviours, do they become the central focus of your life to the point of neglecting important connections such as friendships or family?

17   When you engage in your repetitive sexual behaviours, do they become the central focus of your life to the point of neglecting your important responsibilities resulting in negative consequences to your life?

18   Have you tried to stop your repetitive sexual behaviours?

19   If so, how many times have you tried and failed?

20   When you try, what do you usually do to try stopping?

21   When you have tried, how long have you managed to reduce your unwanted sexual behaviours successfully?

22   When you have tried, how difficult did you find it on a scale of 0–10?

23   What are the negative consequences directly caused by your unwanted sexual behaviours?

24   Have you continued your unwanted sexual behaviours despite the negative consequences directly caused by them?

25   Have you successfully reduced some of the negative consequences directly caused by your unwanted sexual behaviours whilst continuing those behaviours?

26   If so, which negative consequences have you successfully reduced?

27   Do you derive any sexual or psychological pleasure out of your unwanted sexual behaviours?

28   If so, what is the specific pleasure you get from your unwanted sexual behaviours?

29   Is there a particular unwanted sexual behaviour that brings more sexual or psychological pleasure than others?

30   On the scale of 0–10, how much sexual or psychological pleasure do you get with each unwanted sexual behaviour?

31   Do you derive sexual or psychological pleasure from wanted sexual behaviours?

32   How long have you been struggling with your unwanted sexual behaviours?

33   During that whole time, have there been periods of time when it was easier than other times to control your sexual behaviours?

34   During that whole time, has there been times when the unwanted sexual behaviours were non-existent?

35   When were those times?

36   During that whole time, have your unwanted sexual behaviours caused marked distress for you?

37   During that whole time, have your unwanted sexual behaviours caused significant impairment in your life, such as personal, family, social areas?

38   During that whole time, have your unwanted sexual behaviours caused you to stop functioning properly?

39   During that whole time, have your unwanted sexual behaviours caused you to feel bad feelings towards yourself such as guilt, shame, disgust, etc.?

40   During that whole time, have your unwanted sexual behaviours crossed the line to illegal activities?

41   How do you identify your sexual behaviours being unwanted?

42   Do you judge your sexual behaviours based on what you have read in a book or online?

43   Do you judge your sexual behaviours based on what your partner(s) think is acceptable or unacceptable?

44   Do you judge your sexual behaviours based on your values not matching your behaviours?

45   Do you judge your sexual behaviours based on what your religion or faith indicate is unacceptable?

46   Do you judge your sexual behaviours based on being incongruent with your own moral compass?

47   Who disapproves of your sexual behaviours?

48   How do you know what sexual behaviours are wanted and unwanted?

49   Are you able to talk to your sexual partner(s) openly about your sexual desire and arousals?

50   How comfortable are you in a sexual situation?

These enquiries will help clients to begin to unpick their problems in terms of how they think and feel about them. For some clients, these are overwhelming questions so it may be done in several sessions. In between sessions, I sometimes suggest that they keep a diary of their sexual urges so that they can be more aware of their process in mindful observation with these enquiries:

When did I feel an unwanted urge?

How long did it last?

What happened before?

What senses were involved?

What happened afterwards?

What was my emotional state at the time?

How did I feel today? (mind and body)

It is possible that some clients don't meet the criteria for the disorder and also don't appear to have any sexual compulsivity traits. This doesn't mean that all is fine with these clients. Non-consensual non-monogamy is not fine because it is extremely painful and devastating to partners. Most people will feel a lot of remorse for hurting their partner in that way, but not all. How to formulate what is going on for these clients? Some may have low empathy. Some may be neuro-diverse, which makes understanding emotions and empathising with partners difficult. Some men may have some toxic masculinity.

Toxic masculinity

I understand toxic masculinity as men who enjoy dominating others, particularly women, because of a strong belief in misogyny. They tend to promote, or make light of, violence and aggression towards women, including rape. They tend to blame women for their sexual arousal, rather than owning their erotic for themselves. Men with toxic masculinity also tend to be homophobic as their masculinity values are based on strict male stereotypes which reject any sense of tenderness and femininity or same-sex sexual and romantic behaviours. They also particularly become aggressive when someone challenges their views. They are not open to conversations, seeing things from a different perspective or changing their mind.

Since the era of #metoo, a wonderful and much needed movement, I met many heterosexual men who were anxious about having toxic masculinity. Toxic masculinity is very particular. A man who cheats on his partner doesn't mean he has toxic masculinity. A man who is ambitious and puts his career first doesn't necessarily have toxic masculinity. However, a man who prides himself for *'grabbing pussies'*, becomes insulting and aggressive when challenged and is not open to change is likely to have toxic masculinity; I'm sure we can all think of a public figure that might fit this category.

Men with toxic masculinity are also victims of their own tight 'man box' (Hendriksen, 2019). Many of them develop toxic masculinity because they have been socialised from a young age with strict and distorted ideas of masculinity. Those boys and men are taught to:

1   Endure physical and emotional pain in silence.
2   Have no needs for themselves, especially no need for warmth, comfort, love or tenderness.
3   Have no emotions other than bravery and anger. Any emotions might be perceived as weakness. Weakness is absolutely unacceptable.
4   Not depend on anyone. Asking for help is also perceived as weakness. Feeling connected and needing someone else's open arms is also unacceptable.
5   Always win, no matter what, whether it is sport, work, relationships or sex.

Those boys and men are also taught that daring to move out of that tight 'man box' will have dreadful consequences such as total disrespect and a threat of violence from other men, including bullying. These restrictive masculinity messages, which develop into toxic masculinity, is dangerous for those men too because it blunts their emotional awareness. They are not able to detect their emotional distress early enough. They will not ask for help. They are unable to enjoy pleasures in life. They become unaware of others' needs and feelings too, sometimes even mocking others if they express needs. The American Psychological Association (APA) issued their first ever guidelines on working with men and boys in August 2018. The APA reports that men commit 90% of homicides and represent 77% of homicide victims in the United States; and they are 3.5 times more likely than women to die by suicide (www.apa.org). In England and Wales, male suicide represents three-quarters of suicide deaths (www.ons.gov.uk). It is not only men with full-blown toxic masculinity that die by suicide, but, in my clinical experience, the restrictive and distorted ideas of masculinity that are common narratives in our society are so toxic that they infect many men's psyche, their lives and their sense of self. Toxic masculinity harms everybody.

Compulsivity, cheating, accountability

When clients come to their initial assessment because they have been caught, whether the assessment reveals that there may be sexual compulsivity or not, clients may use their therapist's formulations to manipulate what they report back to their partners. Some may say: '*my therapist says I have sexual compulsivity, so it means I can't help myself with these behaviours*'. Others may say: '*my therapist says I don't have sexual compulsivity so I'm fine and you need to change*'. Offering unconditional positive regards and suggesting to clients that they can explore their Erotic Template is not to excuse for their hurtful, betraying behaviours. Clients do need to be accountable for their behaviours, as we all do. They need to acknowledge the hurt they caused their partner and, if they want to repair the relationship, they will need to do much of the hard work to rebuild the trust of their partner. Many people may have non-consensual, non-monogamy behaviours without being compulsive. The drivers for 'cheating' are many and varied, as Esther Perel eloquently explores in her book *The State of Affairs* (2017).

The assessment and treatment explained in this book is appropriate for clients who meet the ICD-11 criteria for the compulsive sexual behaviour disorder, those who don't meet the criteria for the disorder but have some compulsivity issues in their sexual behaviours, those who use other terms to describe their struggles, including '*sex addiction*', '*out of control sexual behaviour*', '*hypersexual*', or '*dysregulated sexual behaviours*'. Although this book focuses on sexual compulsivity, it can also be useful to help clients who have non-compulsive non-consensual non-monogamy behaviours. This book is not for the treatment of sexual offenders.

The sexology assessment

An effective treatment is underpinned by a robust sexology assessment which is framed by a sex-positive philosophy. Based on the relationship between impulsivity and compulsivity (increasing arousal and releasing tension) described in Part 1 of this book, the sexology assessment is to help clients discover their Erotic Template in depth. For this, I borrow the pioneering work of Jack Morin (1995). Some of the central enquiries are:

1   *What are your sexual memories that lead to a peak turn-on?*
2   *What are all the ingredients that makes these memories a peak a turn-on?*
3   *What are your sexual fantasies that lead to a peak turn-on?*
4   *What are all the ingredients that make these fantasies a peak turn-on?*

When I ask these questions, I encourage clients to think about as many details as possible. In my conversations, I weave in enquiries discussed in the Part 1 of this book for a full understanding of all the colours of their painter's palette:

1   The four cornerstones of eroticism
2   The ten erotic boosters
3   The somatic erotic pathways
4   The six principles of sexual health
5   The erotic equation

Slowly, clients can start to piece together their unique Erotic Template. For many clients, it is the first time they can think about their erotic processes free of judgements. This assessment process reduces sexual shame, which is a potent healing agent.

Clients can then assess their sexual behaviours, what is wanted and unwanted through the lens of the six principles of sexual health. Talking about their unwanted sexual behaviours in terms of their breach in their sexual health principles is less shaming and more useful than '*how many times have you watched pornography this week?.*'

Psychosexual problems

In some cases, the sexual behaviours that are incongruent with clients' relationship boundaries may be labeled as sexual compulsivity but it is actually a repeated attempt to resolve basic psychosexual problems such as erectile problems or anorgasmia. Many clients report having good erections with sex workers or watching pornography, but not with their committed partner. The erection problem is not the result of their sexual compulsivity, it is the cause of it as the psychosexual problems often pre-date sexual compulsivity. Unresolved psychosexual problems are often precipitated and maintained by poor sex education or high religiosity.

The most common male sexual problems are:

1   Erectile problems. The difficulty to develop or maintain an erection during sexual activity.
2   Rapid ejaculation. The unwanted ejaculation occurs before penetration or soon after penetration.
3   Delayed ejaculation. The ejaculation is wanted but does not occur after a prolonged time of sexual activity.
4   Male anorgasmia. The wanted orgasm does not occur. This may be linked to delayed ejaculation. Sometimes, ejaculation happens with no pleasurable feelings of orgasm.
5   Loss of sexual desire. There is no sexual desire for their partner or themselves.

The most common female sexual problems are:

1   Vaginismus. Penetration is not possible due to the unvoluntary contracting of muscles.
2   Dyspareunia. Penetration is painful.
3   Female anorgasmia. The wanted orgasm does not occur.
4   Loss of sexual desire. There is no sexual desire for their partner or themselves.

In the context of CSB, these psychosexual problems will be assessed as 'situational', meaning that they only happen under certain situations, mostly with their committed partner, but do not happen with strangers, sex workers, illegitimate lovers, or when watching pornography, hence making the sexual behaviours outside of their relationship boundaries more exciting and powerful. Some clients may describe their sexual problems as 'global', which means that it happens in all situations. If this is the case, the sexual problem could be organic, which requires a thorough medical investigation.

For some people these psychosexual problems may be 'lifelong' which means that client always had the problem. This can be the case when clients describe noticing sexual compulsivity from the beginning of their sex lives. The problems may be 'acquired', usually after a traumatic event. This is when clients describe a good sex life for a period of time and then notice problems starting later on.

It is worth reminding ourselves here of the vast body of research that did not find any evidence of pornography induced erectile dysfunction or any other impact on mental health (Charig et al., 2020). If we make an assumption that sexual problems come from pornography, we might miss much of the important sexology assessment.

The psychological assessment

In the first part of this book I discussed the roles of impulsivity and compulsivity. The impulsivity may indicate a predisposing factor or a precipitating factor of the unwanted sexual behaviours but it does not need to be the point of focus for interventions as it may be quite normative. On the other hand, compulsivity is a maintaining factor. For compulsivity to be established there needs to be a chronic stress. As psychotherapists, it is more useful for us to be curious about what is underneath compulsivity rather than being concerned about impulsivity or trying to stop repetitive behaviours. Assessing the unwanted sexual behaviours that is incongruent with the client's Erotic Template is done through various clinical conversations about their history. The identification of the underlying problems is varied and unique to all. I find it helpful to discuss childhood issues and negative experiences as well as the client's sexual and relational development. Psychotherapists can do this in their own ways. Some therapists may prefer to do it as a timeline exercise. I prefer to do it through guided conversations.

In my experience, the roots of sexual compulsivity may include one or a mix of these factors: unresolved trauma, attachment styles, poor self-esteem, narcissistic traits, a high sexual desire and unresolved psychosexual problems (as discussed in the sexology assessment).

Trauma

Unresolved trauma creates much disturbance in a person's life. It is often undetected if the disturbance is not at Post-Traumatic Stress Disorder (PTSD) level. Often, it is the sexual compulsivity that is a survival strategy against the unresolved trauma, so we should not encourage clients to stop it straight away. Unresolved trauma can become more toxic as time goes on, making sexual compulsivity all encompassing. This is often when people mistake it for an addiction.

Defining trauma is not simple. Different specialists in traumatology offer different definitions. Bessel Van Der Kolk writes:

> trauma, by definition, is unbearable and intolerable. (...) It takes tremendous energy to keep functioning while carrying the memory of terror, and the shame of utter weakness and vulnerability (...) Long after a traumatic experience is over, it may be reactivated at the slightest hint of danger and mobilize disturbed brain circuits and secrete massive amounts of stress hormones (2014, pp. 1–2).

Marich prefers to define trauma more broadly:

> Trauma is a subjective human experience, colored by an individual's perception, life experience, and healing style. My general assumption is

that if an experience is wounding, to a person, we should validate it as traumatic (2014, p. 19).

On the other hand, Levine thinks:

> The healing of trauma depends upon the recognition of its symptoms. Because traumatic symptoms are largely the result of primitive responses, they are often difficult to recognise. People don't need a definition of trauma; we need an experiential sense of how it feels (1997, p. 24).

My opinion is that trauma is subjective and its impact depends on the person's existing coping strategies, so I like to keep in mind all the definitions above. Whatever is your preferred definition, we can all agree that there are four types of trauma:

1 Incidents that threatened the person's life, or were perceived as threatening the person's life.
2 Witnessing acts of violence.
3 Hearing or seeing the death of someone close to the person.
4 Sexual abuse.

Relational trauma

Sanderson expands on our understanding of relational trauma:

> Repeated acts of violence, abuse or humiliation within attachment relationships can have more pervasive immediate and long-term effects due to the aversive dynamics such as betrayal of trust, violation of dependency and protection needs and the severing of human connection, which threatens the sense of self and self-identity (2013, p. 19).

Some of the most painful life experiences are when we get hurt by the very people we love. These experiences are sometimes called 'attachment injuries'.

Symptoms relating to untreated trauma and childhood attachment injuries may range from trauma and stressor-related disorders including Post-traumatic Stress Disorder (PTSD) to difficulties in self-soothing, intimacy and forming good attachments.

Some of the most common symptoms of PTSD include (DSM-5, pp. 271–280):

1 Re-experiencing the traumatic event in a range of sensory forms. This phenomenon is called a flashback.
2 Avoiding reminders of the trauma by avoiding or numbing emotions. In some cases, we call it dissociation.

3 Chronic hyperarousal of the nervous system. This is called dysregulated arousal.

Attachment styles

I am grateful to John Bowlby (1969, 1973, 1980) for gifting us with his attachment theory, as, in my experience, most clients I have worked with have endured varying degrees of attachment disruptions leading to anxious, avoidant or disorganised attachment styles. Someone with a secure attachment does not usually experience sexual compulsivity.

Identifying a client's attachment style is helpful because it can explain some of their choices for attempting to resolve an erotic conflict. Attachment styles harbour subconscious settings that pull the strings of relational and sexual behaviours. They can be compounded or caused by unresolved trauma.

For the purpose of this book, I'm going to simplify attachment theory, to make it most relevant to compulsive sexual behaviours. I fear I will not do any justice to Bowlby's wonderful work and I hope I can be forgiven.

Secure attachment

People who have a secure attachment do well in all types of relationships. They can easily commit to a relationship or relationships. They are often married or partnered in monogamous or open relationships or in polyamory. They are happy and clear about their relational and sexual boundaries. They feel satisfied with what they have, and they tend to have a good level of self-esteem, knowing themselves well. They are able to self-regulate their emotions including stress and anxiety. Their core beliefs sound like: *'No matter what happens to me, there will be people around me supporting me and loving me', 'I know I mess up sometimes but I know I'm a fundamentally decent person'* Therefore, they usually feel safe in their relationships and they are able to tolerate their partners' autonomy. They are not suspicious people as they are trusting of their partners. In the language of Transactional Analysis, people with secure attachment have a life position of: *"I'm OK – You're OK"* (Stewart & Joines, 1987, p. 117). People with secure attachments do not develop compulsive sexual behaviours. However, they may be in a relationship with a partner who is, because their trust can make it easy for the person with CSB to continue their behaviours unnoticed.

Anxious attachment

People with anxious attachment have poor self-esteem. Their core beliefs sound like: *'I'm not good enough'*, *'The world is a bad place'*, *'I'm all alone in the world'*. Their Transactional Analysis life position is: *'I'm not Ok – You're OK.'*

They are desperate for seeking reassurance of connections at all times. They often mis-read their partner's words or body language for rejection as they are sensitive to criticism. In the context of CSB, people with anxious attachment may be married or in monogamous partnership. They may also develop multiple affairs or one long-term one. An affair is a soothing place because the primary focus is on being wanted and desired without all the inconvenience of the daily grind situated in their legitimate relationship. Clients often describe the illegitimate relationship as '*the bubble*'. When they have affairs, they perceive them as a '*safety net*' in case their primary partner leaves them. People with an anxious attachment style may have multiple casual sex encounters. They perceive paying for sex as paying for a connection without any anxiety of rejection or '*I want to be the best client*' to soothe their poor self-esteem. They may use sex workers' services for talking and hugging to soothe the '*I'm not good enough*' core belief. CSB is a coping strategy to manage the consistent anxiety they feel from their primary relationships. People with anxious attachment live in a lot of fear that their partner will stop loving them. It feels too risky for them to address relationship issues with their loved ones.

Avoidant attachment

People with avoidant attachment also have poor self-esteem. Their core beliefs usually sound like '*No matter what happens, I'm alone in the world*'. '*Life is tough*'. '*People are not good*'. Their life position is: '*I'm OK – You're not OK*'. They value their autonomy highly to the point of feeling suffocated or feeling that their space is invaded if a partner comes too close to them. They would often say things like: '*you're too needy*', '*leave me alone*' to their partner. The more their partner tries to talk to them or understand them, the more the people with avoidant attachment want to move away from them and reclaim their independence. In the context of CSB, people with avoidant attachment may be married or partnered in a monogamous or open relationships. Or they may be '*always single*'. They can easily breach agreed boundaries even in open relationships as they often feel suffocated and reclaiming their independence is a priority for them. Their CSB may manifest as multiple short sexual encounters such as '*mini affairs*' or multiple casual sex through apps or paying for sex. People with avoidant attachment tend to have a lot of online sexual behaviours as it is a good way for them to keep their space for themselves. CSB is a strategy for them to escape the suffocation of relationships. It is a way that they remain in control. They manage their stress and anxiety, and any relational angst they might feel with their primary partner(s), by directing sexual feelings and behaviours to others. People with avoidant attachment usually sound like they are only one step away from breaking up with primary partner. With each conflict, big or small, they may automatically think of breaking up and have an exit strategy rather than trying to resolve a conflict. They find it difficult to address problems in their relationships because they're convinced they will be misunderstood so '*what is the point?*'.

Disorganised attachment

People with a disorganised attachment have usually suffered severe trauma in childhood. They fear close proximity or intimacy in relationships. They feel frightened of their vulnerability. They may exhibit extreme rage or anger when challenged by something or someone. They can sometimes lack empathy with others. They have little understanding of boundaries. People with disorganised attachment may exhibit abusive or neglectful behaviours and respond to situations in either frightened or frightening ways. They do not appear to have attaching behaviours. They can often feel confused or apprehensive in the presence of loved ones. Their life position is '*I'm not OK – You're not OK*'. Some people who have a disorganised attachment style are likely to have a narcissistic wounding and therefore they are the ones more likely to have narcissistic traits in their relational behaviours. Their primary goal is to survive faced with their perceived threat, which threshold is usually low. Their moods can be unpredictable and changeable. If their way to stay alive is through sexual behaviours, this will trump any other considerations, including the needs or feelings of their partners. In the context of CSB, they are likely to exhibit the whole range of sexual behaviours outside of their primary relationships, including short and long-term affairs, casual sex, paying for sex and online sexual behaviours. They will do their best to protect their behaviours so they are very good at lying, gaslighting and hiding their behaviours. They usually refuse to go to therapy, or if they do end up in therapy, it is to appease their partner and make them believe they are committed to change when they are not. They will try to make the therapist feel de-skilled.

Poor self-esteem

This is usually one of the main chronic stressors that maintains compulsivity. Poor self-esteem surfaces in different intensities. Sometimes it is undetected, but almost always present. The best way to identify low self-esteem is to listen to client's negative cognition about themselves. Poor self-esteem is usually a result of trauma and anxious, avoidant or disorganised attachment styles. Some clients' poor self-esteem may be increased by poor emotional or psychological health or unsatisfying financial state, lack of intimate relationship or a lack of passionate engagement such as a hobby.

Narcissistic traits

Some clients' sexual compulsivity is maintained by narcissistic traits. Some may have mild traits whilst others may have a more significant narcissistic personality disorder. If sexual compulsivity is a symptom of personality disorder, the treatment should be a specialist personality disorder treatment, not a sexual compulsivity treatment. It is however common for clients to present with mild narcissistic traits, which can be appropriate for sexual compulsivity treatment. It will be addressed with their thinking error on the theme of entitlement and limited empathy. According to Malkin (2015), clients with narcissistic traits are predisposed to it by nature and influenced by the quality of their upbringing, the nurture element. Narcissism usually develops in early childhood, when there is significant trauma which causes an individual to be

> preoccupied with him- or herself to the exclusion of everyone else" and "in denial of feeling", writes (Lowen, 1985, pp. 6, 8).

High sexual desire

Someone with a high sexual desire may perceive themselves to be '*wrong*' or '*bad*' because of messages they might have picked up from childhood or society on how they '*should*' feel or what their sex life '*should*' be. People with a high sexual desire are often seen as 'unhealthy' or 'problematic'. I understand these clients' distress as prolonged sexual shame and the treatment needs to be primarily based on shame reduction. In some cases, high sexual desire may be the result of trauma but it may not always be problematic. For example, some people report managing PTSD with frequent masturbation as their soothing mechanism with no negative consequences. In this instance, it is therefore appropriate, normative and functional, with no need for psychological treatment.

It is impossible to define what is a normal level of sexual desire because there are too many bio-psycho-social factors at play (Bancroft, 2009; Nagoski, 2015; Lehmiller, 2018).

Dr Karen Gurney adds:

> Now we understand that our desire is never static, and we have to remember that we are only really measuring desire in that exact moment (...) our new understandings of desire tell us that it is dependent on context, and so, when we ask about it, we are not learning about the levels of desire within that person but their current desire in that exact moment in that particular context (2020, p. 43).

The moebius loop of shame

The 'sex addiction' literature is concerned with 'the addiction cycle'. I don't think there is such a cycle with compulsive sexual behaviours. However, in my opinion, there is what I call a moebius loop of shame; its toxicity makes the loop seamless and it feels like it is part of people's DNA. The different components of the loop are:

Negative core belief (*'I'm not good enough'*, *'I'm bad, I'm worthless'*, *'I'm unlovable'*). Usually acquired in childhood. (predisposing factor). The Seed of Shame.

Activating event. A difficult meeting with manager. An argument with partner. Erection difficulties. Birth of a child. Completing a big deal at work. Physical pain. The activating event waters the seed of shame into blooming. Negative core beliefs become louder.

Impulsive arousal. Sexual urge to soothe the activating event. It is not a problem in itself if there are many other soothing strategies to choose from. But the CSB population usually don't have other resources. The sexual urges will increase the negative cognition into punishing thoughts (*'I shouldn't feel this way'*. *'I'm a worthless sex addict'*). Shame increases.

Emotional pain. Original negative core belief becomes enflamed, creating more emotional pain, which turns into chronic stress of global thinking about themselves (*'I'm ill'*, *'I'm broken'*, *'I'm defective'*, *'I'm worthless'*, *'I'm a bad person'*, *'I'm unlovable'*). These core beliefs become so loud that it is now impossible for people to hear anything else. Shame is at its most toxic.

The chronic stress and constant toxic shame need to be soothed. As it is chronic, it needs a repetitive solution, which is met by sexual compulsivity.

Unwanted behaviours reinforce the original negative core beliefs, which maintains the chronic stress and toxic shame and completes the loop.

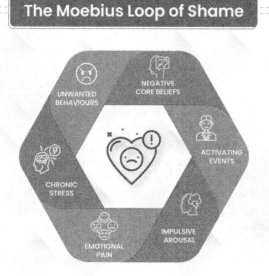

The Moebius Loop of Shame

UNWANTED BEHAVIOURS — NEGATIVE CORE BELIEFS — ACTIVATING EVENTS — IMPULSIVE AROUSAL — EMOTIONAL PAIN — CHRONIC STRESS

When there is sexual compulsivity there is almost always a chronic stress and toxic shame to address. The source of it can sometimes simmer just below consciousness, so it is not always detectable by clients. The process of the psychotherapeutic encounter is to bring the moebius loop of shame to the awareness of the client, safely, and to treat it.

The sexual fantasies and behaviours arising from impulsive arousals to meet the here-and-now chronic stress and toxic shame (precipitating event) may be part of the client's Erotic Template; if so we don't attempt to change it, but we can help clients add more strategies to meet these arousals and urges with tried and tested urge reduction techniques, which I will explain later. When clients have plenty of tools to soothe their toxic shame, the loop is disrupted, they will then naturally be able to self-navigate their lives meaningfully. This is when sexual compulsivity stops.

Identifying maintaining factors: the pie of life

Trauma, attachment styles and psychosexual problems can be both predisposing and precipitating factors of CSB. One of the central maintaining factors of CSB is a poor repertoire of resources with which to manage these problems. These deficits create the chronic stress that demand relief, thus making repetitive sexual behaviours compulsive. When looking at the client's whole life, there is usually a deficiency in several areas. They may have a busy job, but no social life. They may have close friends but no meaningful work. I find that clients like the visual exercise of the pie of life. It helps clients name the areas of their life that are important to them and identify where the gaps are. This exercise is often called the 'Wheel of Life' but I prefer to call it the pie of life because I'm French and a foodie. For me, creating a mindset of abundance disrupts the loop of shame and goes against the process of sexual compulsivity. Using the language of abundance, I usually say something like: 'Sexual compulsivity thrives in deprivation. It tries to compensate for something important that you're not getting. One way to look at it is with your pie of life. Often, many people live a life with one or two slices of their pie, and perhaps a few crumbs from missing slices. That is dissatisfying and keeps you wanting something more. You have the right to have your full pie, consistently. So let's look at the slices that you do have, and those that you need to add for a fuller, delicious pie'.

At the beginning of this exercise, I help clients by naming some of the usual slices that make a good fulfilling pie. In my experience, those slices are: health, work, family of origin or family of choice, friendship and meaningful connections, romantic love, fulfilling sex, passionate engagement, a sense of belonging, finances, a sense of awe. I ask clients if they have more slices that I haven't thought of, or rename some of the slices, so that it becomes their pie. Clients can then begin to think of their life as a delicious pie with many flavours and slices.

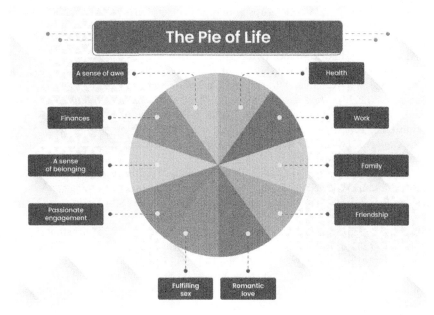

Many clients report their compulsive sexual behaviours are maintained to anaethetise themselves to the feeling of being trapped at work, or loneliness or an existential feeling of not belonging anywhere. These deficits impact on a client's self-concept and increase disturbances. When clients can identify and enjoy all their slices of the pie, they will heal; their sexual behaviours will become congruent with their values: a well-nourished system does not need to resort to compulsivity.

References

American Psychological Association. CE Corner. (2019). APA issues first-ever guidelines for practice with men and boys. [Available online]: https://www.apa.org/monitor/2019/01/ce-cornr.

American Psychological Association, Boys and Men Guidelines Group. (August 2018). APA guidelines for psychological practice with boys and men. Retrieved from http://www.apa.org/about/policy/psychological-practice-boys-men-guidelines.pdf.

Bancroft, J. (2009). *Human sexuality and its problems*, 3rd ed., London: Elsevier.

Bowlby, J. (1969). *Attachment and loss, volume 1: attachment.*, London: Pimlico.

Bowlby, J. (1973). *Attachment and loss, volume 2: separation.*, London: Pimlico.

Bowlby, J. (1980). *Attachment and loss, volume 3: loss.*, London: Pimlico.

Burri, A. (2016). Sexual sensation seeking, sexual compulsivity, and gender identity and its relationship with sexual functioning in a population sample of men and women. *The Journal of Sexual Medicine,* Volume 4, issue 1, P69-77. Elsevier.

Charig et al. (2020). A lack of association between online pornography exposure, sexual functioning, and mental well-being. *Sexual and Relationship Therapy.*

Routledge, 35:2, 258–281. https://doi.org/10.1080/14681994.2020.172787. DOI: 10.1080/14681994.2020.1727874.

DSM-5 (2013). *Diagnostic and statistical manual of mental disorders*, 5th ed. American Psychiatric Association.

ICD-11, International Classification of Disease. 11th revision. *World Health Organisation.* [Available Online]: https://icd.who.int/en.

Gurney, K. (2020). *Mind the gap: the truth about desire and how to futureproof your sex life.* London: Headline Home, Headline Publishing Group.

Hendriksen, E. (2019). How to fight toxic masculinity. *Scientific American. Savvy Psychologist.* [Available Online]: https://www.scientificamerican.com/article/how-to-fight-toxic-masculinity/.

Lehmiller, J. (2018). *The psychology of human sexuality*, 2nd ed., Chichester, West Sussex: John Wiley & Sons.

Levine, P.A. (1997). *Waking the tiger: healing trauma.* Berkeley, California: North Atlantic Books.

Lowen, A. (1985). *Narcissism: denial of the true self.* New York: Touchstone Book.

Malkin, C. (2015). *Rethinking narcissism.* New York: HarperCollins Publishers.

Marich, J. (2014). *Trauma made simple.* Eau Claire: PESI Publishing & Media, PESI.

Morin, J. (1995). *The erotic mind.* New York: HarperCollins Publishers.

Nagoski, E. (2015). *Come as you are: the surprising new science that will transform your sex life.* New York: Scribe Publications.

Office for National Statistics. Suicides in England and Wales (2019 registrations). [Available Online]: https://www.ons.gov.uk/peoplepopulationandcommunity/birthsdeathsandmarriages/deaths/bulletins/suicidesintheunitedkingdom/2019registrations.

Perel, E. (2017). *The state of affairs: rethinking infidelity.* London: Yellow Kite.

Sanderson, C. (2013). *Counselling skills for working with trauma.* London: Jessica Kingsley Publisher.

Stewart, I. and Joines, V. (1987). *TA Today: a new introduction to transactional analysis.* Nottingham: Lifespace Publishing.

Van Der Kolk, B. (2014). *The body keeps the score.* London: Allen Lane.

Chapter 7

The RAW assessment

Throughout the initial, sexology and psychological assessment stage, we have to conduct another assessment; the client's level of readiness, ability and willingness, which I call the RAW Assessment (I'm not a fan of acronyms, but I make an exception for this one). This assessment process will provide plenty of material to figure out how psychotherapists need to pace their therapeutic process, what avenues to explore, which blocks to foresee and to make a prognosis of treatment success. In my opinion, one of the most crucial aspects of good practice is first to assess whether it is right or appropriate for the client to be in therapy in that particular time.

R – ready?

The client's hidden sexual behaviours have just been discovered by their partner. They rushed online to do a test which confirmed they were a '*sex addict*'. They looked through hundreds of therapists' profiles and finally selected you. They made an initial enquiry and a few days later they are in your consulting room for the first time. Making it to that first meeting is not easy. But they turned up. It must mean they're ready, right? They might be ready to seek help. But are they ready to do the work to help themselves? Or are they ready to appease their partner?

Some helpful questions to assess client's readiness are:

1 Is now the best time?
2 How strongly do you want it?
3 Is your goal realistic?
4 Has there been a turning point for you?
5 What is your particular reason for wanting to stop your unwanted behaviours? Is it for your partner? Or is it for you?
6 Does changing your unwanted sexual behaviours matter to you?
7 Are your unwanted sexual behaviours really unwanted if you were being totally honest with yourself?
8 Are there other priorities?

9   Is the goal really desirable?
10 Are you mentally prepared to make some changes?

A – able?

Some clients are not able to engage in the therapeutic process for CSB. It is important to assess the ability as it can be frustrating for the client to be offered a treatment that they are simply unable to follow.

Some aspects of assessment to consider is if the client has an enduring mental health problem that causes symptoms of sexual compulsivity. For example, a client diagnosed with bipolar disorder may have behaviours similar to CSB (McElroy et al., 1996). In such instance, it is best to refer the client to a specialist in bipolar disorders rather than offering a CSB treatment.

Borderline personality disorder or narcissistic personality disorder may not respond to CSB therapy as the therapy requires a significant level of introspection which is a common difficulty for people with such diagnoses. According to the DSM-5 (2013) one of the diagnostic criteria for borderline personality disorder is 'marked impulsivity' (2013, p. 663). One of the traits of narcissistic personality disorder is 'a sense of entitlement' (2013, p. 669). These two components may show up in people with CSB. If in doubt, I recommend referring clients to a clinician specialised in personality disorders for a second professional opinion. If the client is diagnosed with one of these personality disorders, they would do better to have a long-term psychological treatment focused on that rather than a CSB treatment. Similarly, people who have active psychosis often have CSB symptoms but are best cared for by psychiatrists in the first instance.

Some neurological medical conditions can bring CSB symptoms such as dementia, head trauma, cerebral anoxia, multiple sclerosis, Parkinsonian disorders and other brain diseases (Mendez and Shapira, 2013). Sexual compulsivity symptoms were found to be mostly pronounced in people with behavioural variant frontotemporal dementia (Black et al., 2005). It is obviously not appropriate to offer a treatment for CSB to these populations.

W – willing

How long does a new year resolution last? Why is it so hard for people to change their diet permanently? Think about how difficult it is to break a habit and to establish a new one? We, human beings, do not like change. We feel safe in patterns of behaviours even if we know that they create problems.

When we first meet a client with CSB, we often meet someone who is in great distress, they can appear desperate to change, but desperation does not make someone willing to change. Some of the questions I ask are:

Is the behaviour change worth it? What is it worth? Why?
Does the behaviour change have value to you?

As most people are not willing to change so easily, one of the important strategies from the beginning of therapy is to boost the client's intention by focusing on their attitudes to their desired outcomes, whilst informing them of what is achievable and what is not. Clients often say:

I want to stop watching pornography forever
I want to only have sex with my husband and nobody else
I want to stop cheating on my wife
I want to stop masturbating in secret

These statements are desperate statements but not words of willingness. I encourage them to think differently: *'I hear what you want to stop doing. But what do you want to start doing?'*

As I mention several times in this book, the language of abundance is more helpful for clients than the one of deprivation. Eliciting clients' hopes goes a long way towards successful therapy.

Pros and cons of change

The therapeutic space needs to be established as a safe space from the beginning to encourage honesty. Shame and guilt will stop clients telling the truth. It is the rights of clients to hide some truths or to lie to their therapists. There is a therapeutic value in clients admitting their lies later. As soon as our space is set up as the therapist in the *"Parent Ego State"* (Berne, 2009), an easy set up if we're not careful, then the therapy is likely to be unsuccessful. The fertile therapeutic space is one when the therapist can open conversations with their clients about not wanting to change, hence, the importance of the conversations about the pros and cons to change.

Clients might say:

Pros/gains: 'I will feel less stressed because I won't have to hide my phone all the time'.
Cons/sacrifices: 'I will miss the buzz of getting a sexual text from my casual sex partners'.
Pros/gains: 'I will have more time to focus on my children'.
Cons/sacrifices: 'It will be hard to give up feeling sexy when I meet my casual sex partners'.

The therapist needs to be willing to hear the gains and sacrifices of change from the clients with an absolute unconditional positive regard in order to make the therapy safe for clients, both in *'Adult Ego States'*.

Praise

If we are too keen to praise clients for stopping a behaviour we can un-knowingly set up the *'Parent/Child Ego States'*. In the therapeutic context, giving praise can therefore be unhelpful. Here is an example of a helpful exchange instead:

Client: *'I have deleted the hook up app'*
Therapist: *'What did you do to make it happen?'*
Client: *'I have started to read a really good book and it's a positive distraction from thoughts of checking people for casual sex'*
Therapist: *'How do you feel?'*
Client: *'I'm pleased with myself'.*

Tracking change

How and when?

Clients can track change with a diary, recording their urges, emotions, what happened at the time, and what they did to manage it. Some clients opt for a quiet time of self-reflection or mindfulness either on a daily basis or weekly basis.

By whom?

Tracking change should never be done by the client's partner. It is unfair on the partner to bear the responsibility of their loved one's sexual behaviours. It sets the couple up in the *'Parent/Child Ego States'* which would be a disaster for the couple. Tracking change is best done by clients themselves. Indeed, good CSB therapy is one when there is no suggestions from the therapist to stop sexual behaviours.

Setting goals

Goals should be SMART (Specific, Measurable, Appropriate, Reasonable, Time-limited). They should be affirmative too.

Specific: rather than *'I will stop watching pornography forever'* opt for: *'This week, I will watch pornography from 7.30am until 8am, to give myself time to get ready for work'.*

Measurable: rather than *'I will delete my hook up apps'* opt for: *'I will delete my hook up apps on Monday and monitor how I am feeling with my stress level and my urges three times a day. I will use my helpful resources to manage any difficult emotions and I will review how it is going the following Monday'.*

Appropriate, Reasonable and Time-limited: rather than '*I will be sexually sober for 90 days*' opt for: '*This week, I will help myself staying away from sex workers by engaging with my sexual thoughts and feelings through masturbation only. I will review at the end of the week*'.

Goals should be set in small steps. Therapists can normalise resistance and explain that it is just feedback. The therapist can help the client think of their self-reward: for example: '*I deleted the hook-up app so I'm going to indulge in a really good and pleasurable activity like reading a really good book*'.

The traffic lights exercise

Clients often find helpful to have a visual representation of their goals. I introduce the traffic lights exercise when clients have a clear idea of their Erotic Template as well as the behaviours that are outside of their painter's palette, values and integrity. I usually start with the green light.

Green: Sexual and romantic behaviours clients want and need as part of their erotic and relational life. The green section needs to be full and rich incorporating all the elements of their painter's palette they have discovered in their sexology assessment.

Amber: The sexual or romantic elements they are unsure of, or the ingredients that needs more exploration before figuring out whether it goes in the green or the red. The Amber section can also be the areas that are in erotic conflict with their partner(s).

Red: The sexual and romantic elements that they absolutely do not want in their erotic or relational life. These need to be only what is outside of their Erotic Template and it must not be informed by partner's disapproval, but only by the client's own values, integrity and their commitment to their partner(s). The elements that breach the six principles of sexual health is a good guide to know what needs to be in the red section.

It is important to tell clients that their traffic lights exercise is not set in stone and should be revisited on a regular basis as they progress in their therapy and find new meaning.

The therapist's RAW assessment: self-reflection

When we assess a client, we have to assess ourselves too. Are we suitable to work with the client in front of us?
Ready?
Am I ready to work with this client?
What is my workload like?

Do I have enough energy and space to take on a new complex client?

Do I have enough training and knowledge on human sexuality for this particular client?

What would I need to do to expand my knowledge?

Do I feel confident working with the client?

Is there something that bothers me about them?

Can I resolve it with myself?

Do I need to speak to my supervisor?

Some therapists choose this field of work because of their own past struggles with compulsive sexual behaviours. If this is you, you have to be extra careful not to project your own path onto your clients. It is important not to prescribe to them what had worked or didn't work for you. Are you ready to be curious about your client's Erotic Template? Are you comfortable being curious about your own Erotic Template?

Able?

What is going on for me currently?

Am I truly able to be fully present with the client?

Am I truly able to offer unconditional positive regard?

If a client presents with some extreme sexual behaviours that you find difficult to hear, are you able to be present? If not, what would you need to be more able? My CSB therapy approach focuses on exploring sexual behaviours. It means that you will need to dive in detail into the erotic world of your clients. Are you able to do so with clients who identify as kinky, or BDSM? Do you need further training on these topics?

Willing?

Perhaps you have all the skills and knowledge to work with a new client, but you are not willing. If you have a long caseload of clients with CSB, you might not be willing to work with another one. There is nothing wrong with that. In fact, it is an important consideration to remain the best therapist you can be to the clients you already have.

Assessments as short-term therapy

If you work in the NHS or in an organisation that offers limited amount of sessions, you may not have enough time to do the full treatment approach described in this book, but it may be enough sessions to help clients explore their Erotic Template and their emotional story that led them to their sexual compulsivity. These assessments are therapeutic for clients. If clients finish their short-term therapy with a much better understanding of their Erotic Template, they may start to make some meaning of it, which would be a great outcome for the short time together. Don't underestimate the power of human connection in meaningful conversations.

References

Berne, E. (2009). *Transactional analysis in psychotherapy*. California, USA: Snowball Publishing.

Black et al. (2005). Inappropriate sexual behaviours in dementia. *Journal of Geriatric Psychiatry and Neurology*, 18(3), 155–162.

DSM-5. (2013). *Diagnostic and statistical manual of mental disorders*, 5th ed. Washington, D.C.: American Psychiatric Association.

McElroy et al. (1996). Are impulse-control disorders related to bipolar disorder? *Comprehensive Psychiatry.*, 37(4), 229–240.

Mendez, M.F. and Shapira, J.S. (2013). Hypersexual behavior in frontotemporal dementia: a comparison with early-onset Alzheimer's disease. *Archives of Sexual Behavior*, 42(3), 501–509.

Wells, A. (2009). *Metacognitive therapy for anxiety and depression*. New York: The Guildford Press.

Chapter 8

Client stories
Assessment and formulation

I will introduce you to clients, amalgams of people I have worked with from across the spectrum of gender, sexuality and relationship diversities. All identifying information has been changed to protect confidentiality and permission has been given to share these amended stories.

Heterosexual men

The heterosexual male CSB population comes with great diversity of sexual behaviours. Here, I will present two cases that are common presentations. However, remember that some men who self-identify as heterosexual will present with some same-sex behaviours, and many will say that they are attracted to transgender people or cross-dressing, for example, which brings up much shame for them. For those clients, the CSB assessment and treatment process is the same as the following case studies.

Roger

Roger was a 43-year-old cisgender, heterosexual man. He came to me one week after his wife Megan discovered his hidden sexual behaviours. He had been married for twenty years and had two teenagers. He worked in a high-pressure employment where he held a post of great responsibility for decision making. Whilst he was successful in his career, he had been compulsively visiting sex workers for the entirety of his marriage. Megan did not consent to non-monogamy. Roger reported that he loved Megan and there was nothing wrong in their relationship, yet, he felt compelled to visit sex workers. He did not understand why.

Roger's greatest current distress was to face the possibility that Megan might leave him.

Exploring his Erotic Template, Roger discovered that his peak turn-on was having sex with Megan, missionary position, connected with eye contact. The ingredients were giving sexual pleasure to her, feeling like a good lover, feeling like a man, the smell and touch of her skin, and the sexual sound that Megan made when having intercourse. His erotic boosters were touch, scent and sound. Roger said that sound was the most dominant of the three. These peak-turn-on memories seemed to be congruent with his sexual behaviours with Megan. When we discussed the pleasurable aspects of his visits to sex workers, he described something surprising; the most arousing moment for him was when the door opened and he was let in by the sex worker, rather than any of the sexual aspects of the behaviours. He described being accepted into the intimate world of another as the most potent. There were many different colours in the palette of his Erotic Template. Being desired by Megan was 'risky' because he loved her, so he felt a lot of pressure to be perfect for her. He feared that if he showed flaws, she would leave him, which indicated an anxious attachment style. With sex workers, he was able to freely enjoy being desired without the emotional risk of being left.

Roger was shocked to realise that he breached most of the principles of sexual health. He felt he achieved mutual pleasure with Megan but he questioned it with sex workers as it was essentially a transaction. One of his fantasies was the hope to be the best customer for them. Exploring his Erotic Template and the breach of his sexual health principles empowered Roger to think about what neuroscientist Marc Lewis eloquently describes as 'the realignment of desire' (2015, p. 208).

His childhood stories were full of parental neglect and violence. He had never told most of those stories to anyone else. In fact, he had come to believe that it was a 'normal' childhood. At birth, Roger's mother was disappointed; she wanted a daughter because her first born was a boy. She encouraged her son to beat Roger up. On many occasions, Roger was left unconscious after a beating. He thought that one day, his brother would kill him. His mother frequently punished him and beat him up too, whilst his father passively watched. The pieces of our assessment started to make a coherent picture for Roger; it made sense that he harboured a subconscious script of 'I'm all alone in the world'. His anxious attachment became normalised as the impact of such childhood leaving him with a bruised self-worth, feeling he was not good enough to love. He started to understand the erotic arousal of sex worker visits; being invited inside an intimate space where his needs would be looked after. Roger's unwanted and repetitive sexual behaviours served the purpose to get what he had longed for in his childhood: unconditional love, an attempt to repair trauma.

Roger's somatic erotic pathways were identified with two factors, when he felt bad about himself (something went wrong at work); and when he felt good about himself (he completed a great project at work). His problematic sexual behaviours were for both soothing and celebrating himself; two processes he had never learnt to do as a child.

He identified that there were deficits in his pie of life because he was overworking. He now understood that it was another way to heal his bruised self-esteem. Another maintaining factor that kept his compulsive system intact was his self-defeating beliefs. Roger's distorted beliefs sounded like 'Megan is probably faking her orgasms', 'Megan doesn't really love me', 'Megan is bored with me', 'I'm a pervert', 'I'm worthless'. Birchard calls these thinking errors as 'name calling and self-blame' (2015, p. 76). Roger started to acknowledge that he needed to face his self-hatred, which he inherited from his childhood experiences, and which kept him in his loop of toxic shame.

Martin

Martin was a 25-year-old cisgender man who self-identified as a 'porn addict'. He accessed pornography and masturbated to it compulsively several times a day for several hours each time. It left him with little time to meet his needs in the other areas of his life. He decided to seek therapy because his behaviours had a negative impact on his life: his relationship with his girlfriend Amy was fragile as he kept pushing her away so that he could have some 'alone time' with pornography. He was self-employed and lost significant income to the point of financial difficulties for watching pornography instead of working. Martin decided to seek therapy when he masturbated so hard that his penis was injured with blisters. He then continued to masturbate and made the injury worse.

His girlfriend Amy was open-minded about pornography and did not put pressure on him to stop. Martin attempted to stop watching pornography, once by himself and once with the help of a 12-step group. Both failed.

Martin was unable to identify peak sexual memories. He described all of his sexual memory experiences as 'all right' and anxiety provoking. He found his peak sexual fantasy turn-on, however, hard to choose, given the range of pornography he was watching. He finally identified his peak sexual fantasy turn on as a 'gangbang', where one woman would enjoy having sex with several men. The ingredients that made this a turn-on were specific: a blond, curvy woman looking into the eyes of men as they climaxed inside her. Martin explained that these were the kind of images he searched for on the internet as they were the ones that usually made him ejaculate. As he usually spent hours online looking for 'gangbang' videos, I enquired if he also enjoyed the practice of edging as part of his turn-on. He never thought about that before but he agreed. Edging, a practice of masturbation that keeps the level of sexual arousal on the edge of climax, was then identified as his peak sexual memory turn-on. From the psychosexual problems perspective we hypothesised that sexual intercourse with women may not be so satisfying because he had now trained his penis to feel sensations with the hard grip of his hand that couldn't occur with vaginal intercourse.

Martin thought there was an issue in his sex life with Amy because he felt awkward having sex with her. Looking at his erotic history, he identified that he'd always had sexual anxiety. He breached the sexual principle of honesty as he divulged that he never told Amy about the specific things he liked sexually. Similarly, he never asked her what she liked. It wasn't surprising that there was anxiety with sex with Amy ... he was in the dark!

Martin identified the starting point of his pornography and masturbation behaviours when he was 10 years old. It started when his mother died. It was a shocking sudden death in a car accident. His father was very upset but didn't discuss any of it with Martin. There was an unspoken rule that it was forbidden to bring her up in conversations, so Martin kept all of his thoughts and feelings about her death to himself. Martin spent hours alone in his bedroom at a time when he discovered masturbation, which he found helped reduce his intense emotions for a while and helped him sleep. Soon after that, he discovered that he could watch pornography on his computer for an unlimited time as his father was absent. Pornography and masturbation became a fascination for Martin because it was the only thing that took him away from his emotional pain. As the years went by, pornography and masturbation became his primary way to engage with his sexuality and to soothe all of his emotions. The source of his sexual urge dysregulation was his unprocessed grief.

During the exploration of Martin's Erotic Template, I opened a dialogue about the possibility of digisexuality. Martin could relate to it but he also expressed a longing to have sex with Amy without anxiety, therefore he identified that there were some digisexuality colours on his painter's palette, but they were not a dominant part.

Martin's loop of shame started with the negative core belief: '*I'm going to be abandoned*' and '*I'm not worthy of love*'. Immediately after ejaculating, he would feel bad about himself with thoughts like '*I'm one of those porn addicts*', '*I'm a wanker*', which reinforces the story '*I'm going to be abandoned*'. Also, he compared himself to porn stars: '*if only I had a bigger penis like them*', which brought hopelessness, a pervasive emotion that contributed to his chronic stress that needed consistent soothing.

Women

Female sexuality is largely shamed because our society is uncomfortable with it. Women who have a high sexual desire or who choose not to have children are frowned upon. Not too long ago, women were pathologised with the diagnosis of 'nymphomaniac' if they dared having too much sexual desire. In our modern time, the label 'nymphomaniac' is commonly replaced by 'slut', which is equally damaging. McKinney (2014) reminds us that female 'sex addiction' presentations are quite absent in the vast literature on this subject, sometimes added as an after-thought. She looks through the lens of the feminist's perspective to see that female hypersexuality is a social construct made by males which creates a major block in understanding female sexuality. According to Covington, women who benefited from the 'sexual revolution' and are able to be assertive with their rights are still facing the difficulty of socialisation in the sexual space where the concept of the split of "*Madonna/Whore*" is still apparent and "*still operating on a deep level*". Covington also highlights the societal conditioning on women and their pleasure as not being important or even desirable; having sex means bringing pleasure to their partner, but not seek their own sexual satisfaction. Women have vibrant sexuality as much as men, they are capable of objectifying and have casual sex just like men. Because of the social stigma, they may not always come to therapy and admit to casual sex. Livingstone perfectly sums this up:

> Women's stories of problematic sexual behaviours are hidden, obscured by dominant narratives about female sexuality that conceptualise them in derogative ways (...) I believe their conflicts reflect the profound difficulties women can face in trying to 'realise' themselves in a complex, contradictory, patriarchal social system (2017).

McKinney (2014) points out that there is little literature on the influence of father/daughter attachment bond compared to the mother/son one, yet, the role of the father seems to be a central part of the attachment disturbances leading to sexual compulsivity for women. I agree with this. In most of my female clients, we found a history of paternal neglect. The typical stories I hear are either fathers being cold and emotionally absent or abusive or overprotective and controlling. McKinney goes on to explain other factors such as trauma and insecure and disorganised attachment as important factors to female sexual compulsivity.

Francesca

Francesca, a 33-year-old cisgender woman, met many men each week, flirting with them first with the aim of '*manipulating them into falling in lust with her*'. She identified this to be a pattern she had followed for many years. It felt compulsive to her. She recognised she ended with her being hurt and not getting what she wanted. Ultimately, she wanted to be loved in a stable relationship.

Francesca particularly enjoyed making married men forget about their wives, this was highly erotic for her. The sexual activity part of her compulsive sexual behaviours was not as potent as the chase and the manipulation. She used the term 'manipulation' because she wasn't honest with the men she pursued. She invented a character only for the purpose of seduction. The most potent ingredient to her peak turn-on was the cornerstone of eroticism 'searching for power'.

Her peak-fantasy turn-on was what she called a '*fairy tale*'. Seducing a man who would be crazy about her and then marry her and live happy ever after. Although she knew it was a fairy tale, she enjoyed refuging to that fantasy often as it was a good antidote to stress. The most potent ingredient to this was '*total acceptance*'. She identified her erotic booster as when she heard men say to her that she's the best lover and she '*drove them crazy*'. During sex, she would often engineer this kind of comments by asking them: '*do you like it?*' '*I bet you've never felt so good*' '*is your wife as good as me?*', and so on. She recognised that she was breaching the sexual health principles of non-exploitation, honesty and shared values by being a fake character to lure men. She knew it was impossible to create a genuine long-term relationship when starting off with a fake character. She vowed to herself many times that she would stop doing it, but she never actually tried to stop.

She was sexually and psychologically abused by her father from the age of five to ten. At the time, she feared him and she loved him at the same time. She felt she had no control over his behaviours, she could only submit to his moods. She had to please him so that he wouldn't be upset with her. She was silenced, her father repeatedly said to her: '*we have a special bond that most people don't understand. If you tell anyone what we're doing, you will be sent to an orphanage*'. She feared that consequence, and she complied with his demands. Her mother lived with them, but she was oblivious to the abuse as she was often drunk. When she was thirteen, her father left the household without any warning. Francesca felt abandoned and betrayed by him. Her mother fell apart at that point, drinking even more. All of this happened behind closed doors and was undetected because she was very good with her schoolwork. She learnt how to play fake characters then.

Together, we identified her attachment style as avoidant. Her core belief was '*I'm OK – You're not OK*'. It brought some clarity into her underlying constant bubbling anger that informed her erotic booster.

In the here-and-now, she was successful in her career, but her life felt empty. She didn't have any long friendships. Her fridge was mostly empty, apart from frozen peas in her freezer. She didn't take good care of herself. Her pie of life was in major deficit, apart from work and money. Controlling men was a way to soothe her childhood trauma, therefore the fantasy and the trauma were the two different faces of the same coin.

The assessment period was tricky. She would often miss appointments and then ask if I could waive my late cancellation fee for her. I did not. She would get angry, sometimes raising her voice at me. Our conflictual conversations were an opportunity to discuss boundaries in relationships and her need to feel special by having me make an exception with my policy. Wasn't it a parallel process with her trying to feel special by getting men to breach their monogamy agreement with their spouse? It was difficult for Francesca, but she took the challenge and gradually she engaged in therapy with less late cancellations.

Anna

Anna was a 31-year-old cisgender woman who self-identified as heterosexual and polyamorous. She was in a sexual and romantic relationship with three men who self-identified as polyamorous too. They did not live together. Sometimes they would meet separately and sometimes together. Outside of her primary relationships, she enjoyed going to sex clubs where she could meet her sexual needs with casual partners. Her peak turn-on with sexual encounters in sex clubs was to be dominant. She enjoyed the preparation to wear specific gear, usually PVC with knee high boots. She would sometimes wear a long wig, and she enjoyed using objects such as a whip. The peak element was to be someone different from her everyday life, and to feel powerful towards other men, especially men who would look dominant but had a submissive turn-on. The peak turn-on of sex with her three primary partners was the opposite, it was when she could be herself, being known really well by them, truly seen. Communication between them could be non-verbal and she could relax. She called it her 'Haven'. She liked that her three partners were open-minded sexually and happy to try new things. All of these arrangements were consensual between all parties involved. She did not experience any distress from her sex life in her twenties but things changed when she turned 30. She was in a good career trajectory in a law firm but felt she had to steer away from conversations about relationships with her colleagues who were mostly heterosexual and monogamous men. She told me that she already felt scrutinised because her success 'intimidated men', she thought that if someone found out about her relationship and sexual life, they would trip her up and destroy the career she worked so hard for. As she reached 30, she described noticing a change in other people's attitudes, conversations about 'settling down', 'getting married', and 'having a baby' became more frequent. Anna felt great discomfort with these conversations because she did not relate to any of them, but also she felt these conversations were increasingly imposed on her, by both her male colleagues and her female friends. She started to feel bad about herself because she realised she was losing friendships, one after another. When her friends started to settle down and have babies, there was no more space for other conversations or connection with them. Anna thought that there might be something wrong with her as she kept hearing her friends saying: '*I didn't want a child in my twenties, but in my thirties, something changed, I really wanted one, because it is nature and it is the most wonderful thing a woman can do*'. Anna had never felt that way. The thought of having a child or settling down with one person felt completely alien to her. Her male colleagues started to scrutinise her more as it became more and more obvious that she would avoid all conversations about having a family. Although her three partners reassured her that she was loved and nothing was wrong with her, she believed them less and less. She stopped enjoying sex both with her primary partners and with casual partners because she could not be in the moment anymore, the thought *'something is wrong with me'* took hold of her. She started to feel depressed about it and she wondered if her poly-amorous and kink orientations meant that she had sexual compulsivity. Was feeling no desires for children an anomaly? Was it against nature? Was she fooling herself for believing that her sex life was ok? This is when she made the call to see me. She described her childhood as 'privileged'. She was an only child in a middle-class family. There was no pressure on her to be a particular way. They were both proud that she found a good career for herself. She didn't tell her parents about her relationships and they did not put pressure on her to discuss private matters.

Gay men

Working with gay men involves a thorough understanding of the impact of heteronormativity. The environment in which the LGBTQ+ population lives is full of prejudice, discrimination about their sexual orientation and stigmatisation of their sexual behaviours, which creates what is called minority stress (Meyer, 2003). Minority stress has the impact of:

1. Experiencing prejudice about their sexuality
2. Expecting rejection
3. Hiding their sexuality
4. Negative thoughts about their own sexuality (internalised homophobia)
5. Changing their instinctual behaviours to fit with heteronormativity as a coping strategy

Davies and Neal explain:

> It is important to examine one's ideas about values, morals and lifestyles when working with clients who are culturally different. It is probable that most lesbian, gay and bisexual clients are unlikely to share the lifestyle of their therapist, especially when she or he is heterosexual. There are a wide variety of lifestyles enjoyed by lesbian, gay men and bisexuals. Some live in relationships almost identical to heterosexual married couples, or very different (2011, p. 27).

Joe Kort's definition of Gay Affirmative Therapy (GAT) is an essential framework when working with gay men, and all other populations within the LGBTQ+ minorities:

> the position that there is nothing inherently wrong with being LGBTQ. What's wrong is what is done to LGBTQ individuals by homophobic, homo-ignorant society and heterosexist therapy. Living in a shame-

based culture creates a variety of behavioral and psychological disorders. GAT focuses on repairing the harm done to these clients,
helping them move from shame to pride (2018, p. 21).

Peter

Peter was a 40-year-old cisgender gay man. He was in a monogamous relationship with his husband Carlos for four years. Previously, he had described himself as promiscuous but in control of his sex life. Now that he
was in a monogamous marriage, he felt out of control as he seemed unable
to keep to his monogamous arrangement with Carlos. In the four years of
their relationship, Peter consistently met with other men, mostly strangers in
sex clubs, without Carlos' consent. Peter reported his monogamy-breaching
behaviours were of weekly frequency. He came to see me because he feared
he was a 'sex addict' and he wanted to stop his compulsive unwanted sexual
behaviours before Carlos discovered them.

Peter described his sexual memory peak turn-on as being when he first
arrived in London after growing up in rural Wales. He remembered feeling
intensely sexually aroused being in Soho amongst many other beautiful gay
men. One of his first sexual encounters happened in the dark room of a club
when he felt the sexual touch, smell and breath of men touching him whilst
being surrounded by others having sex. The ingredients that made this a
peak sexual turn-on memory were the sense of unknown and danger and the
abandon into pure hedonism that he understood as total acceptance of his
body and sexuality. He also remembered the smell of many male bodies and
the sexual sounds mixed with hard music, an arousing combination for him.
He described it as the feeling of being '*on the top of the world*'. This became a
strong somatic erotic pathway for him. When recounting this memory Peter
described it as '*intoxicating*'. He reported getting sexually aroused in my
consulting room.

His peak sexual fantasy turn-on was to live as a nudist with two or three
other gay men. I pointed out to Peter that his sexual fantasy sounded like a
relational desire. Peter took some time to think about it and the relationship
between his fantasy, desire and monogamy.

Peter described violating prohibition as a major cornerstone of eroticism
for him. It was partly going against rural Wales where only heterosexuality
was visible. It was partly going against the rules of society, having group sex
in sex clubs was not the image of a '*good boy*'. In sex clubs, he enjoyed letting
'*men take him*'. He described that he could let himself go, feeling joy with no
worries in the world, enjoying his body to the maximum.

Peter's erotic booster was mostly kinaesthetic. He said that every part of
his body was erogenous. He loved being touched, which is one of the reasons
he enjoyed group sex so much. He also enjoyed the visual, olfactory and
auditory erotic boosters. The hard music, the smell of poppers, the smell of

male sweat, watching others have sex with each other, hearing men moan with pleasure, were all very highly erotically potent for Peter. Discussing all of Peter's Erotic Template, he started to wonder if he was a man who naturally had a high sexual desire.

There was an erotic charge in the consulting room especially as Peter expressed feeling aroused whilst talking about his peak sexual memory turn-on. Peter mentioned that he chose me as a therapist because he made an assumption that I was a gay man after reading the content of my website and my professional Instagram profile. Later, he disclosed that his type of men was 'Mediterranean', the physical description that can be attributed to me. Him feeling aroused whilst sharing the '*intoxicating*' element of his erotic memory was a way to feel close to me. I entertained the hypothesis of internalised homo-negativity with which Peter may mis-direct his eroticism onto me in believing that every gay man is sexually available. Peter's sub-conscious sense of my '*knowing*' and my '*holding*' to be his companion on his path without losing his own autonomy was a parallel process with submitting himself to men in sex clubs whilst remaining in control.

It was hard for Peter to talk about exploiting his relationship with Carlos with non-consensual non-monogamy, but he accepted it, with sadness. Protection from STI was a difficult topic too. He looked after his sexual health by having regular check-ups but he was aware that he practiced sex without condoms. Although he protected himself from HIV with PrEP, there was a high risk of contracting other STIs which he could easily pass on to Carlos as they were sexually active. Luckily, he had consistently tested negative on all STIs. He lived with a lot shame and guilt for exposing his husband to such risks.

Peter said he didn't have erection problems but Carlos was penis focused. He would always reach for Peter's penis as an invitation for sex and he felt bad if his penis wasn't instantly hard enough when he touched it. He wished his husband could focus on other parts of his body when initiating sex. Peter had never had this conversation with Carlos, which meant that there was also a problem with honesty and shared values.

Peter's pie of life seemed to be in deficit. His sexual activities pre-occupied him so much that he didn't have time for much in his life apart from work and spending some time with Carlos. The rest of the time was spent thinking about sex with others. One of the most puzzling elements for Peter was that he never felt a sense of belonging. He had some limited beliefs: '*that's what gay men do*', '*it's impossible for gay men to be monogamous*', '*what Carlos doesn't know won't hurt him*', '*it's only sex*'. These beliefs kept him in the compulsive system. Many gay men are stuck in the moebius loop of shame and live with internalised homo-negativity as Downs honestly describes in his book *The Velvet Rage*(2012).

When Peter was 7 years old he played with his sister's barbie doll, his father saw him and scolded him. He was not to do so again. He then remembered that his father talked a lot in homophobic terms. Peter felt he had to hide his sexuality throughout his childhood '*acting more manly*' than he naturally was. He also forced himself to have a girlfriend at the age of fifteen because it was what his father and his Welsh community had expected. Peter had always thought of his childhood as '*normal*' but now that he thought about it, he realised that the atmosphere was consistently cold and disapproving. Peter felt he had to hide in order to keep the love of his parents.

Some of his internalised homo-negativity is reflected in his cognitive patterns when talking about gay men in a global way: '*all gay men are promiscuous*', for example. Internalised homo-negativity is a powerful disturbance that turns shame toxic.

Chemsex

Chemsex is the term coined by David Stuart currently working in one of Europe's busiest NHS sexual health clinics, 56 Dean Street in Soho. Chemsex is used to describe a sexual behaviour amongst men who have sex with men (MSM) under the influence of psychoactive drugs, primarily mephedrone (GHB), butyrolactone (GBL) and crystal methamphetamine. These drugs are often taken to facilitate sexual activities lasting several hours and, sometimes, days with multiple sexual partners.

George

George came to see me on a Tuesday when he was on a come-down from the previous weekend. He decided to make an appointment with me because one of his friends died of an overdose. Although he didn't want to die like his friend, he found it impossible to stop his drug use.

Mephedrone and crystal meth are stimulants increasing the heart rate and blood pressure, producing euphoria and sexual arousal. GHB and GBL are psychological disinhibitors and mild anaesthetics. Taking the combination of these drugs therefore increases sexual arousal and reduced inhibitions. The unspoken rule of these private parties, also called 'chill out parties', is that nobody discloses their HIV status and it is assumed bareback sex is the preference.

The Chemsex Study (Bourne et al., 2014) looked at the relationship between Chemsex and sex, relationships and intimacy. It supports the psychological evidence that Chemsex is not only a drug problem; it is a psychosexual and a relational one. It is maintained by difficulties with intimacy, self-esteem, self-worth and body image. It is rooted in internalised homo-negativity and it is governed by deep-seated negative core beliefs about self.

Chemsex behaviours may have many negative consequences in people's lives, including a high rate of HIV transmission, although these have decreased since PrEP became available to buy. In the come-down stage, people often feel intense shame, they are angry at themselves, disgusted, depressed, anxious and physically ill. *The Chemsex Study* reports:

> Many participants described how drugs could significantly increase sexual desire or libido, but at the same time diminish sexual performance. Erectile dysfunction under the influence of crystal meth and mephedrone was very widely reported, as was retarded ejaculation (2014, p. 43).

The use the of drugs also has severe consequences in other areas of people's lives including keeping jobs, friendships, romantic relationships, loss of physical health and ultimately death. Hammoud et al. (2018) found that overdose was more likely with frequent GHB use.

The hidden epidemic of Chemsex

The Chemsex drugs are cheap and easy to access, and the geo-location apps make it easy to be invited to private parties. The combination of these factors contributes to the prevalence of the hidden epidemic of Chemsex amongst gay men and MSM. After repeated Chemsex use, people often report being unable to have sober sex.

Why is Chemsex so popular amongst gay men and MSM? Engaging in sexual activities can be tricky for everybody. It brings up the anxiety of being rejected. For gay men and MSM, these anxieties are more intense because the gay culture puts sexual potency on a pedestal. There is so much pressure to be '*perfect*'. Of course, the fear of rejection and the perfection desire of the gay culture exist for a good reason; it is a coping strategy to ward off the sense of vulnerability as a community because of so much past trauma of the ostracisation of gay people, the criminalisation and the pathologising of homosexuality. Today, we are still living in a world where more than 70 countries have laws against homosexuality, according to the Human Dignity Trust. We can understand why Chemsex drugs can appear to be the antidote to so much existential angst. With Chemsex, there is an instant sense of connection, no rejection, no criticism of body image, sexual performance or age, everybody is welcome and everybody can enjoy their right of having sexual pleasure with no shame and no restriction. In his provoking book *Unlimited Intimacy* (2009), Dean proposes that the bareback community may thrive on total acceptance; a pure equalitarian community where all is welcome to access sexual pleasure.

George had strong internalised homo-negativity. The more George swore to himself that he wouldn't do Chemsex on the weekend, the more he failed to keep his own promise, the more he believed that he was '*broken*'. George started to interact only with people who also did Chemsex. It was not until I enquired about the quality of these friendships that George realised he didn't actually know them very well. His world became small; his pie of life was crumbs.

George wasn't sure if people had sex with him when he was too unconscious to consent. He wondered if he had been exploited on several occasions. He wasn't sure if he paid attention to shared valued as he would do some sexual things outside of his boundaries.

Within our therapeutic relationship, his anxious attachment played out. He wanted me to be a '*sorted, married therapist living in a big house*' because it was something that he aspired to, but at the same time, he felt so broken that he could never reach it, so he used the same aspiration to push me away; being that therapist meant I wouldn't understand him. Yet, if I was a therapist enjoying drugs and sex clubs, it wouldn't feel stable enough for him.

The Chemsex journey

Although there are many negative consequences to Chemsex the popularity of it indicates that there are some significant gains too. As clinicians, we must understand these gains to have a balanced view and to see clients who struggle with Chemsex as whole. Smith and Tasker (2018) revealed that Chemsex was associated with a positive gay identity gain which makes it hard for them to stop the behaviours. The study describes a spiralling effect starting with positive experiences, thus creating a somatic erotic pathway. When aided with the drugs, there is less inhibition and less fear of rejection, so their sense of self identifying themselves as gay men can become more meaningful. As they continue to explore their sexuality further, the cornerstones of eroticism come into play. Many gay men will enjoy the violation of prohibition and search for power by pushing back boundaries. The Chemsex drugs can relax people's bodies to the point of pushing the boundaries of sexual explorations further, for example, experimenting with fisting. There is no denying that the popularity of Chemsex is partly due to the fact that people enter in a relationship with the drugs quickly, it provides them with a space for exploring sexual pleasure and deepening their sense of identity and intimacy.

Power et al. (2018) argue that there might be more positive aspects of Chemsex. Their study reveal that some people feel a better sense of connectedness within their community, including their subculture, which helps with feeling safer from the outside world that still stigmatises HIV positive status people. Of course, we know that having a sense of belonging and connection with our peers increases wellbeing. When clients come to us wanting to stop Chemsex behaviours, they are not only asking of themselves to stop taking some drugs, they are facing a significant loss of a meaningful space in which they found a sense of belonging.

The dual process of the deliberative and affective system is evident with clients struggling with Chemsex. They know that it is bad for them, yet the emotional pull may impair their decision making.

George couldn't identify specific memories where his parents were overtly homophobic, although there was most definitely a strong sense of what was expected: good grades, dating girls at the appropriate age and doing boys activities. George said that he felt misunderstood. He noticed his father preferred his brother because they were both into football, and George wasn't. This was his first taste of conditional love. His mother was mostly critical. He experienced her as cold and unloving. He kept most of his emotions to himself, especially the fear of being abnormal for liking boys. When he became a teenager, he dated a girl to hide his sexuality. Going to University was a good excuse to break up with her, he felt guilt about it. George went to study in a city far away from home where he didn't know anybody and where there was good LGBTQ visibility. He felt he didn't have to hide anymore and wanted to embrace his sexuality. However, he quickly realised that he felt as awkward amongst his peers as he did with '*the straights*'. He was now struggling to be intimate with others because he developed strong negative critical thoughts about himself. Going to a gay bar sober was intensely stressful for him. He didn't want to be seen as a '*country bumkin*' by all the sophisticated city gay men. He imagined that everybody would reject him. Before long, he met people in the Chemsex scene where same-sex connection was offered to him on a chemical platter.

Chemsex assessment: asking the right questions at the right time

As with all compulsive sexual behaviours, therapists have to be mindful to avoid setting up a power dynamic of approving clients' sobriety goals. Stuart cautions us with his "*golden rule*" (2014):

> Refrain from using terms like 'addict', 'addiction', 'drug abuse', and 'drug misuse' (drug use is preferable). It may be challenging for us as health workers to see self-harmful behaviour, but the golden rule of substance use work is to keep the client engaged.

Assessment questions have to remain open and non-judgemental, incorporating the general compulsivity questions mentioned earlier, as well as enquiries about safer Chemsex use.

Chemsex care planning

Stuart and Weymann (2015) offer a guide on creating a Chemsex care plan with clients which should be to identify small and realistic goals, based on when they are most vulnerable to their Chemsex urges. George had his strongest urges on Friday night because it was the weekend. We brain-stormed together; how about visiting a friend for one weekend, instead of doing Chemsex? I stressed that these goals are 'experiments' to check how he was getting on rather than goals that must be successful. I reassured him that if goals aren't reached the experience can still be valuable as an opportunity to learn more about our processes. No failure – only feedback.

Queer population: kink community

Many people in the communities of Gender Sexuality Relationship Diversity (GSRD) call themselves Queer. It was originally a derogatory term when used by heterosexual people to insult GSRD people, but had been reclaimed by the GSRD communities. The Queer community easily embraces their non-binary self, their mix of masculinity and femininity, more than those who self-identify as gay men. They enjoy their own expression of art and fashion and have established a rich culture of their own.

Kink and fetishes are not to be pathologised in our sex-positive philosophy. Some may identify their kink and fetish as a sexual orientation. We don't make assumptions that BDSM practices are trauma-based, as discussed in part 1 of this book, as there is no evidence that BDSM or kink is caused by trauma (Shahbaz and Chirinos, 2017).

BDSM and kink can be as valid a colour in a person's painter's palette as any other sexual activities or turn-ons. Some heterosexual people may have some kinks and fetishes that are not typically seen as heterosexual behaviours. Although this is a section on Queer population, some of the assessment and interventions may be appropriate to the kink heterosexual population too.

Pascale

Pascale self-identified as pansexual, Gender Queer and a vagina-owner. Their pronoun was 'they/their'. Pascale was French who was aware that their good looks made flirting with both men and women easy. They practiced BDSM. Shibari (roping) as submissive was the peak turn-on for them. They usually preferred one-to-one sex sessions with partners who were experienced in Shibari and whom they knew well. They enjoyed long, un-hurried sessions on weekends. For them, their sex life was an event, with much preparation, discussions and action. They described these events as being 'at peace' and 'at home'. From their first teenage sexual experience, they knew that they weren't vanilla. However, there was a part of their sexual life that Pascale became concerned about. They didn't feel they could talk about it with their peers because of shame. For about one year, Pascale's sexual behaviours started to change; they started to meet strangers, and asked to be punched, cut and strangled. Pascale couldn't feel their body anymore. They couldn't feel any pleasure through masturbation either. They described their body as being 'dead'. It was puzzling to them. In the attempt to feel something, they started to deviate from the three pillars of BDSM (safe, sane, consensual) and stopped making sure they were safe, there were no more negotiated safe words. At the time, Pascale was unaware that one couldn't consent to self-harm thus breaching their sexual health principles. As a result, they attracted some people who weren't from the BDSM community but were sadists. In one encounter, they thought that the man they invited in their home might have wanted to kill them. They stopped just in time, but Pascale could see in the man's eyes that he wanted to do some permanent harm. Other times, the encounters were so violent that it took Pascale several days to recover, sometimes having to take time off work and sometimes feeling a lot of pain. On the one hand, they didn't mind the pain because it was the only time when they could feel their body. On the other hand, it was concerning to them.

We made sure we didn't pathologise their BDSM practice and made the clear differentiation between their safe, sane and consensual BDSM practices to the unwanted sexual behaviours that distressed Pascale. To make the differentiation even more pronounced, I asked them if they wanted to call the concerning behaviours a different name from BDSM. They paused for a moment, to try to find the term that fitted. They came up with an interesting and dark phrase '*Violent rape*'. In French, this translates as '*viol violent*'. Pascale called it '*poetic*', whilst smiling, because 'violent' was half of the word 'rape' ('viol'). Their tone was light and humorous, it was a discrepancy between the subject of the conversation and the observable mood. I asked them if they felt they were being raped when engaging in the unwanted sexual behaviours. They said '*no*' then added '*but I suppose people looking at it would think so*'. I was curious at what precipitated the unwanted sexual behaviours after years of a flourishing and rich sexual life that remained within the sexual health principles and within the Shabbaz and Chirinos Heathy BDSM Checklist (2017). When I asked Pascale about their childhood, they could hardly remember anything before the age of 15. They couldn't remember any trauma or any unpleasant memories. Usually, when there is such a lack of memory, I hypothesise that there might be a trauma that both mind and body are trying to protect a person from. If they were to remember it, they might become so overwhelmed that they would fall apart. One of the trauma therapy principles is to avoid such events so as not to re-traumatise clients (Rothschild, 2000, 2010, 2017). I thought that Pascale was describing dissociation. I didn't say this to them straight away, because I wasn't yet sure, and I never assume or imply to a client that they suffered a trauma when there is no memory. Because of major memory blanks, we couldn't talk much about the past, but we talked about whatever we could, safely. I was watching closely for any trauma activation with every single word they spoke.

Although Pascale said their sexual behaviours changed gradually, there was a clear difference from one year to the next. They recollected that they had no problems with their sex life until it started to change in 2012, and became what they described as 'out of control'. They could not understand why as there was nothing that they could identify as precipitating factors, no anniversaries, no significant events. They described what they could re-member of their childhood as 'fine'. They explained that they were 'privi-leged' coming from a wealthy French family. They said that their parents were 'fine' but emotionally distant. They had two siblings, one who became a drug addict and was constantly in and out of expensive rehab, the other died by suicide a few years ago. They said this with no affect. I asked them how they felt about their brother's suicide. They responded with *'it is what it is'* in English. I pointed out to them that they switched to English, was it harder to talk about it in their mother tongue? They shrugged their shoulders and said *'of course not. I switch languages sometimes'*. I noticed that conversations with Pascale were easy when we talked about their erotic mind. However, I perceived them to be much more guarded when talking about their childhood. Pascale's answers became short statements, they didn't appear as curious as I was.

People of religious beliefs

Different religions will have different sexual prohibition and relational prescriptions. Some of those may not fit with our Western philosophy. For example, in the UK we do not promote arranged marriage or polygamy. We have values against misogyny, and we uphold the human rights of women accessing abortions. However, despite the laws, many people live their lives by the rules of their religion. It is crucial as psychotherapists that we do not shame such clients because of their choice of religion. If we, therapists, are atheists, we need to remain with our clinical opinion of investigating the impact of some religious teachings on sexual dysfunctions, whilst honouring and validating clients' religious beliefs. If we share the same religion as our clients, we need to be mindful of our blind spots, and how we might collude with some unhelpful messages that maintain sexual dysfunctions. Psychotherapy is a profession of self-reflection, all of us, religious or not, must keep in touch with our own internal processes and our blind spots.

In the context of compulsive sexual behaviours, people with religious faith are particularly vulnerable to sexual shame from their own judgmental thoughts, but also from their religious community. They might often feel hopeless and helpless and they could be at high risk of suicidal ideation.

It is particularly difficult for LGBTQ+ people who have a religious faith to 'marry' the two. Jaspal writes about the difficult conflict that Muslim MSM face:

while homosexuality has increasingly gained social acceptance in the UK, it remains highly stigmatised in Muslim societies. Some British Muslim MSM reportedly feel that they are viewed by other Muslims as being 'too British' (that is, as having assimilated the norms and values of British society) due to their sexual identity. This can make some individuals feel like less 'authentic' Muslims, potentially problematising their religious identity. On the other hand, British national identity can sometimes act as a buffer against threat. For instance, some individuals may reject the perceived 'Islamic stance' on their sexual identity and, conversely, embrace the 'British stance', which is perceived as more readily accommodating sexual diversity (2018, p. 119).

Some people living in the UK live in fear of the threat of death if they were to deviate from what is imposed on them under their religious or cultural dogmas. It is important that we, therapists, are alert to these for safeguarding purposes.

Terry

Terry came to see me because of 'pornography addiction'. He felt compelled to watch pornography and masturbated three times a day, when the opportunity arose, which was usually once in the morning, once at lunch time in the toilets of his work, and once in the evening when his family was asleep. Terry was a devout Christian. He told me that his porn and masturbation behaviours were unacceptable for him to do, yet he was unable to stop by himself. He made an appointment with me because his wife, Claire, caught him watching pornography the previous weekend. He was distraught that he caused so much pain to her, it was completely against their religious values. Claire didn't know the full story. Terry revealed to me that his *porn addiction escalated to more sin*'. Last month, he met with a sex worker. He said to me that he had only done it once. He also said that he had regular non-sexual massages with masseuses in secret. Terry thought that if his wife found out about the sex worker, it would be an instant end to his marriage and he was convinced that she would ostracise him from his beloved Church community. Terry's sense of 'wrongness' was activated by acute shame.

I stressed to Terry that the treatment I offered would not be about repressing his sexual behaviours, nor blaming his religion or his wife, but to understand his multi-layered erotic conflicts and the incongruence between his sexual behaviours and values. Some clients of religious faith sometimes decide not to take my offering and seek a therapist willing to offer them a programme to 'stop acting out'. I do not want to persuade clients to do therapy with me. I respect clients' autonomy. I'm happy for clients to disagree with me and find help elsewhere.

Terry watched what he called '*the normal stuff*' in pornography, meaning a man and a woman performing penis in vaginal penetration. What he loved the most was when he could see the '*money shot*' (i.e.: ejaculation) on the exterior, usually on the woman's large breasts. He didn't know why this was so arousing for him. His favourite pornography performers were women with super large breasts who were '*hypersexed*'. Seeing a woman with much sexual desire is erotically potent for him, mostly because it was out of his ordinary. Terry and I discussed that watching pornography was a window to his erotic mind. He said that the hypersexed women and large breasts was more fantasy-based and he didn't want it in his own sex life. However, he would like his sex life to change.

Terry became sad as he described not having had much sexual exploration in his life. He grew up in a devout Christian family, met Claire within that community and got married pretty quickly. They were one another's first sexual partner. They lived the '*perfect and pure romance*'; two young sweethearts, losing their virginity to each other, getting married, having children, being good citizens'. Now, Terry was in his early 60's, their children had left home, and he felt he never gifted himself with the opportunity to explore his sexuality properly. He said with tears in his eyes '*I don't think we ever had a good sex life*'. He did have many memories of sexual excitement watching pornography and masturbating, although they quickly followed with the feeling of shame. I told him that these memories were the memories of good sex with himself. He hadn't thought about that but he accepted the re-frame.

When Terry began to explore his Erotic Template, he noticed feeling sexual attraction for Claire, a feeling he hadn't felt in a long time. He realised that he wasn't attracted to the performers in pornography but he wished his wife could be more embracing of sexuality.

Violating prohibition was a source of eroticism for Terry. Women were not supposed to be super sexual. Sex should be '*nice*', '*clean*' and '*romantic*'. The problem was that these things did not arouse him; he thought something was wrong with him. He hadn't had sex with Claire for two years. He had no indications that she was sexual in any way, they never talked about it. Terry became honest with himself and faced his reality; he found Claire attractive but her attitude was a turn-off.

Terry found it easy to identify his erotic boosters. The more obvious one was visual. There was a strong emotional component to his booster because the sexual attitude of women is an integral part of his Erotic Template. By contrast, he described Claire as not enjoying sex with him. The thought of trying to have sex with her now brought up a lot of dread. From Terry's point of view Claire appeared to endure it, which was a breach of mutual pleasure. His pornography watching, masturbation and his visit to the sex worker were secrets in breach of their shared values and honesty.

Terry lived in an enormous erotic conflict between his Christian values and his Erotic Template. He wanted to stay married to Claire. His Christian faith was very important to him. His erotic self was also important to him.

Terry described his childhood as *'calm and shielded'* with two loving Christian parents. However, there were clear messages about sexual prohibition and a strict prescription of masculinity; men were supposed to be strong, non-emotional, and leaders. As a child he was reprimanded for showing emotions, and he had to *'pull himself together'* quickly. The understanding of his anxious attachment was helpful for Terry to examine because it brought clarity to him on how he conducted his marriage with Claire. Rather than blaming her for not initiating sex, what was his part in not upsetting the apple cart?

Terry's pie of life was mostly full. However, his moebius loop of shame was strong and tight. Any sexual feelings, fantasies, thought, longing, yearning produced a strong sense of shame. Negative cognitions automatically surfaced: *'I'm bad', 'I'm wrong', 'I'm a sinner'*, which produced rumination about his 'defectiveness'.

All in all, Terry did not have a significant history of psychological disturbances or trauma, although not being soothed by parents could be perceived as a relational trauma.

References

Birchard, T. (2015). *CBT for compulsive sexual behaviour.* Hove, East Sussex:Routledge.

Bourne et al. (2014). The Chemsex study. *Sigma Research: London School of Hygiene and Tropical Medicine.* ISBN: 978-1-906673-19-2. Downloaded from: www.sigmaresearch.org.uk/chemsex.

Covington, S.S. (1997). Women, addiction and sexuality. *Co-director, Institute of Relational Development*, in L. Straussner and E. Zelvin (Eds), *Gender issues in addiction: men and women in treatment*, Jason Aronson.

Davies, D. and Neal, C. (2011). *Pink therapy.* Maidenhead, Berkshire, England: Open University Press.

Dean, T. (2009). *Unlimited Intimacy. Reflection on the subculture of barebacking.* Chicago: The University of Chicago Press.

Downs, A. (2012). *The velvet rage.* Boston, MA: Da Capo Press.

Grubbs et al. (2020). Moral incongruence and compulsive sexual behaviour: results from cross-sectional interactions and parallel growth curve analyses. *Journal of Abnormal Psychology*, 129(3), 266–278. doi: 10.1037/abn0000501.

Hammoud et al. (2018). Intensive sex partying with gamma-hydroxybutyrate: factors associated with using gamma-hydroxybutyrate for chemsex among Australian gay and bisexual men – results from the Flux Study. *Sexual Health*, 15, 123–134.

Human Dignity Trust, [Available online]: https://www.humandignitytrust.org/lgbt-the-law/map-of-criminalisation/?type_filter=crim_lgbt.

Jaspal, R. (2018). *Enhancing sexual health, self-identity and wellbeing among men who have sex with men: a guide for practitioners.* London: Jessica Kingsley Publishers.

Kort, J. (2018). *LGBTQ clients in therapy: clinical issues and treatment strategies.* New York: W.W. Norton & Company.

Lewis, M. (2015). *The biology of desire: why addiction is not a disease.* New York: PublicAffairs.

Livingstone, S. (2017). Women at the edge. *Therapy Today Magazine* (May), 24–27.

McKinney, F. (2014). A relational model of therapists' experience of affect regulation in psychological therapy with female sex addiction. Article in the Middlesex University's Research Repository. Downloaded from: https://eprints.mdx.ac.uk.

Meyer, I.H. (2003). Prejudice, social stress, and mental health in lesbian, gay, and bisexual populations: conceptual issues and research evidence. *Psychological Bulletin,* 129(5), 674–697.

Morin, J. (1995). *The erotic mind.* HarperCollins Publishers.

Moser, C. (2016). Defining sexual orientation. *Archives of Sexual Behaviours,* 45, 505–508.

Power et al. (2018). Sex, drugs and social connectedness: wellbeing amongst HIV-positive gay and bisexual men who use party-and-play drugs. *Sexual Health,* 15, 135–143.

Rothschild, B. (2000). *The body remembers: the psychophysiology of trauma and trauma treatment.* New York: W.W. Norton & Company.

Rothschild, B. (2010). *8 keys to safe trauma recovery: take-charge strategies to empower your healing.* New York: W.W. Norton & Company.

Rothschild, B. (2017). *The body remembers, volume 2. Revolutionizing trauma treatment.* New York: W.W. Norton & Company.

Shahbaz, C. and Chirinos, P. (2017). *Becoming a kink aware therapist.* New York: Routledge, Taylor & Francis.

Smith, V. and Tasker, F. (2018). Gay men's chemsex survival stories. *Sexual Health Journal,* 15, 116–122.

Stewart, I. and Joines, V. (1987). *TA Today: a new introduction to transactional analysis,* Nottingham: Lifespace Publishing.

Stuart, D. (2014). Sexualised drug use by MSM (ChemSex): a toolkit for GUM/HIV staff. *HIV Nursing,* 14(2), 15–19.

Stuart, D. Website, [Available online]: https://www.davidstuart.org.

Stuart and Weymann (2015). ChemSex and care-planning: one year in practice. *HIV Nursing,* 15, 24–28.

Twist, M.L.C. and McArthur N. (2020). Introduction to special issue on digihealth and sexual health. *Sexual and Relationship Therapy,* 35(2), 131–136.

Part III

Pluralistic treatment for compulsive sexual behaviours

Chapter 9

The three phase treatment approach

As I discussed in previous chapters, each client has their unique Erotic Template, psychosexual elements and their psychological processes. Therefore, treatment of CSB will be different with every client. I will explain my three-phase protocol model to treat compulsive sexual behaviours. The treatment should not look like it is phased, though; it is a careful craft where the wholeness of the client is at the centre, every part of the client can be seen, informed by and addressed with every modality. It is the responsibility of the psychotherapist to integrate and embed the pluralistic knowledge in a seamless process for the client. The psychotherapeutic relationship is an ongoing intervention, which needs to start from the initial consultation. In my three-phase treatment method, I would like you to think more about these phases being intertwined rather than linear; every moment of direct psychological contact with the client is an opportunity for positive change. The three-phase protocol is not my invention. It is borrowed from the field of traumatology, originally invented by Pierre Janet and resurrected by the famous trauma therapist Babette Rothschild (2017). Following Rothschild's steps, I have adapted it for the treatment protocol for CSB.

1 **Phase 1: regulation (impulse control):** Emotional regulations and stabilisation, including managing urges.
2 **Phase 2: reprocessing (treating compulsivity):** Treatment of the identified disturbances underlying compulsivity. Trauma therapy (if necessary). Relational and psychotherapeutic process. Sex therapy (if necessary). Processing client's life story.
3 **Phase 3: reconstruction (meaning-making):** Reconstructing their lives with a reality-based narrative, including a thriving sex life, through meaning-making and existential processes.

In my clinical experience, this structure seems to be optimal for helping people with CSB.

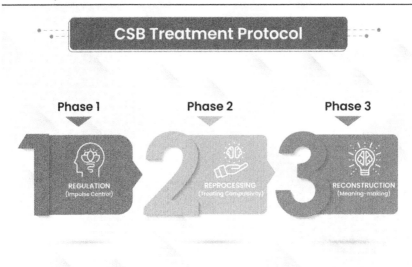

The pluralistic lens

When one therapeutic modality window seems too narrow to understand the client, you can then look through another window and see what the view is from there. The main psychotherapeutic modalities I use to treat the underlying causes of sexual compulsivity are: Psychosexual Therapy, Gestalt Therapy, Cognitive Behavioural Therapy (CBT), Psychodynamic Therapy, Transactional Analysis (TA), Acceptance and Commitment Therapy (ACT), Dialectical Behavioural Therapy (DBT), Person-Centred therapy, Somatic Trauma Therapy, Eye Movement Desensitisation Reprocessing (EMDR) and Emotional Freedom Technique (EFT), all within the humanistic and relational frame.

Do not fear, you don't need to be an expert in all of these modalities, nor do you need to use them all. As long as you keep the sex-positive frame and your robust grounding in sexology, all psychotherapeutic modalities that you are already trained in will help with Phase 2. As a true integrative psychotherapist, I don't believe there is one modality superior to another. However, I do recommend you have specific psychosexual knowledge and are trauma therapy informed.

Erotic transference and countertransference

When we psychotherapists offer a connection-focused treatment, we will inevitably encounter erotic transference and countertransference given that these phenomena are very much about connection. Psychotherapists need to be fully aware of their own erotic self, so that they can safely enrich the therapeutic work when they encounter the client's erotic transference. In this line of work it would be a missed opportunity if the therapist avoided unpacking their client's erotic transference and the potential erotic countertransference as part of an in-depth exploration of the client's Erotic Template in relation to others. The avoidance usually comes from the therapist not being comfortable with the sexual content or their own sexuality. If the therapist is fully erotically processed and has a robust grounding in their sexuality, there should be no anxiety nor reluctance to explore clients' erotic transference and their countertransference. I feel concerned when I hear therapists say that they never identify these phenomena in their work. I wonder what the therapist dis-owns. The main concern for me is that when the therapist dismisses their own erotic, they are at greater risk of harming clients, in two ways:

1   They become subconsciously seductive with their clients, using the client's material for their own erotic curiosity, and potentially leading to inappropriate sexual conversations or behaviours towards the client.
2   They shame the client for labelling an erotic charge in the consulting room as 'objectifying' or 'sexualising' them in an attempt to get rid of something that the therapist can't hold for themselves.

I talked about it in Part 1, but let me repeat myself: I believe it is imperative for therapists choosing to work with sexual compulsivity to adopt a sex-positive philosophy and be erotically well processed (Luca, 2014).

References

ICD-11, International Classification of Disease. 11th revision. World Health Organisation. [Available online]: https://icd.who.int/en.

Luca, M. (2014). *Sexual attraction in therapy: clinical perspectives on moving beyond the taboo – a guide for training and practice.* Chichester, West Sussex: Wiley Blackwell.

Rothschild, B. (2017). *The body remembers, volume 2. Revolutionizing trauma treatment.* New York: W.W. Norton & Company.

Chapter 10

Phase 1: Emotional regulation

Impulse control

Starting the treatment with emotional regulation is how therapists can help clients with their impulse control. When clients struggle to manage their emotions or their urges, they can get in the way of the deeper thinking required for Phase 2. In my clinical practice I have identified three broad circumstances for emotional regulations and impulse control:

1 Emotional regulation for urge reduction.
2 Emotional regulation for shame reduction.
3 Emotional regulation when faced with partner's upset.

Emotional regulation for urge reduction

Clients' unwanted repetitive sexual behaviours will often be their only resource to manage their emotions because of poor impulse control. This phase helps clients add more resources to manage their urges and their life. We must not take away any of their existing resources including their unwanted sexual behaviours. When clients feel more confident with new and diverse resources, the CSB resources become less compelling thus urges become less intense and less frequent over time. Clients can learn to understand their sexual urges and fantasies and surf them, rather than trying to avoid or endure them, or feel overwhelmed by their impulses. Some of the most popular resources are:

1 Mindfulness
2 Multiple Awareness (awareness of the here and now as well as the past and future)
3 Muscle toning
4 Soothing object
5 Anchoring
6 Internal Safe place
7 Support network outside of therapy (external safe place)
8 Meaningful connection

At the beginning of their therapy, I often hear clients ask me if they should put a block on their phone to stop them from accessing pornography or sex workers' sites. I question what they would learn about themselves if they did so. Relying on the external locus of control like a block (or a Higher Power) isn't effective in the long-term because it doesn't help them learn anything. Besides, we live in a world where sex is all around us, whether it is an advert for chocolate or the big billboards of half-naked super models. Living in avoidance is a joyless life. I challenge my clients to learn to access their internal locus of control instead, because this will be more useful and these skills will last a lifetime. I believe that by encouraging clients to find new emotional regulation techniques is to give them the great gift of self-care and autonomy.

Mindfulness

All of us can find an example of our thoughts quickly spiralling into rumination and worry from an activating event. Many people struggling with sexual compulsivity say their sexuality has *'gone out of control'*, but it is often their thoughts that have gone out of control. The antidote to stop our thoughts from getting out of control is, paradoxically, to try to stop controlling them by practicing mindful observation. It sounds like this: *'I saw an attractive person in the street. Even though I'm on my way to the office, I'm feeling horny right now. I'm enjoying this deeply human and exciting experience with myself and I will continue walking to my office to be ready for my meeting'*. Mindfulness is popular now. There are many apps that are helpful to guide clients such as *HeadSpace* or *Calm*. I do caution clients and therapists that the point of taking up mindfulness is for emotional regulation but not to become mindfulness masters. If clients are interested in pursuing full mindfulness programmes, that is great, but it is not essential for effective emotional regulation.

Multiple awareness

Our brain is amazing. We are capable of multiple awareness. We can be in our living room in the here-and-now and we can also find ourselves on a beach, just with our imagination. Spending some time helping clients to be conscious of their multiple awareness does a lot of good for mind flexibility. In the middle of an urge, it feels like there is no multiple awareness; people are fixated on that one thing they want to do. This is actually the mind being in the past memory of the sexual pleasure they felt with that particular activity, possibly through a somatic erotic pathway. With mind flexibility, clients can start to recognise that their strong urge is about one awareness and they can learn to find the awareness of the here-and-now. For example: *'I have a strong urge to masturbate because I remember how good it feels from past experience. I want to do this in the next minute. But, right now, I am here, breathing and feeling the urge'.*

Muscle toning

This is a good technique when the urges are so strong that it is almost impossible to think. Clenching fists tightly whilst counting to five and releasing slowly and counting back to one is a simple technique that helps get back into the here-and-now and thereby reducing urges. If clients are at their work desk and they don't want to be seen doing fist clenching, they can do the same with their feet, going on tiptoe and going on their heels feeling the muscles involved in these movements.

Soothing object

Clients can identify an object that they can easily carry with them at all times so that they can touch it in moments of strong urges. It may be a pendant, a ring, a soft ball in the pocket, the image of someone or something on their phone screensaver that they associate with calm, joy or wellbeing. By making contact with that object, the emotional energy changes and the urge can reduce and disappear.

Anchoring

As well as an object, clients can learn to anchor themselves in various ways. For some, it may be to think of a happy and joyful image. It may be to smell an essential oil they love. It may be touching a part of their body that represents anchoring for them, for example, they may want to touch their chest. Putting slight pressure on the sternum with one finger (also called the Heart Centre) has a calming effect. To some extent, we all touch a part of our body quite naturally when we experience difficult emotions. I'm sure we've all seen people tapping on their temples in moments of stress. But not everybody is fully conscious of their automatic anchoring.

Internal safe place

Our brain can transport us anywhere we want in less than a second. This is partly why we have urges, our brain can take us to a place of pleasure, to avoid pain. With the same great wonders of our brain, we can transport ourselves to places of joy, contentment, peace and calm. The beauty of this is that it doesn't even have to be a real place. We can create our own to make it just right for us. The internal safe place needs to include all of our senses. Once clients have a very good internal safe place, they can add several others, because they may not always want to be in the same safe place all the time. This exercise, in itself, is a classic method to help with impulse control.

Support network outside of therapy (external safe place)

Compulsive sexual behaviours bring up much shame, it can be isolating. Often clients will have nobody to talk to honestly about it but they will be faced with a tremendous amount of intense emotions when they start this work and seeing their partner hurt. It is crucial to identify with clients who they can call for support in between sessions. You might have guessed that I do not recommend a 12-step fellowship as a support network. Clients may identify a good friend whom they think would be non-judgmental and supportive, but also not collude with their behaviours or blaming their partner. Men, especially, need to hear the psychological message: *'it's ok not to be ok'* and *'it's ok to talk'*. I invite client to do what I call the Connection Circles exercise. Clients can look at all their connections and put them in various circles; the inner circle of connection is where they have their most loved ones and best friendships, and a wider circle with good friends and another wider circle with friends for fun but not as meaningful, to the outer circle of connection where they may have acquaintances, or colleagues. In the inner circle, they can include pets; they are an under-rated yet important source of connection. We can help clients identify other support they may want to access, for example going to a weekly mindfulness class or a yoga class could be a great point of regular support, where they are around people doing the same activity but not necessarily talking about their problems. These points of support may be identified as the external locus of control, but by choosing which one they need at any given time means that they are also exercising their inner locus of control. If clients feel urges late at night when support networks are less available, I suggest they can write a letter to me and bring it to the next session. The process of writing can help with self-regulation too.

Meaningful connection

Following on from the Connection Circle exercise, clients can then check if they want to move some people that had drifted to the wider circles, closer to the inner circle. Often I hear clients say that they had lost touch with very good friends. It may be a good time to reconnect. They may also decide that someone in their inner circle isn't actually very helpful or supportive. They can decide to move that person to a wider circle. Therapists can guide clients with thinking for themselves about who they want in their inner circle as opposed to who they think they '*should*' have. Feeling connected to good people is a good grounding element even if these people aren't available at the time, just thinking about them can reduce an urge.

Meaningful interests and passionate engagement

This is one of the most common deficits seen in a client's pie of life. Meaningful interests and passionate engagements help us connect with ourselves. Clients often say: '*I used to have a hobby but I haven't done it in years*'. In this case, there is no need to look further. You can ask clients what it would be like to reconnect with their lost hobby. When they do so, they reconnect to a part of themselves that they like, where they can find some joy and passion. Having this conversation is a way to give clients the permission to do something they had always wanted to do but never taken the time to do, for example, doing a wine course, or learning a new language. Having compelling interests and passionate engagement can help bring meaning to one's life. As I wrote in Part 1 of this book: compulsivity doesn't survive in meaning. The more a client finds meaning in their life, the less compulsive they become.

Better work and life balance

People with CSB will often see in their pie of life that there is a major work and life imbalance. For some, it is not working enough, and for others it is working too much. Both of these will create the significant chronic stress that CSB serves to soothe. It is important not to make assumptions though. Working 'too much' or 'not enough' is subjective to the client and it depends on how they feel about it. For some people their work is their passionate engagement and meaningful interest, working for many hours may not be a place of stress for them. When clients say that they're overworking for a company that makes them feel bad, this is when you might help the client address their work and life balance. The therapist's consulting room is a place where clients can give themselves the time to think and embrace their own sense of agency and decision making. When clients start to re-configure a life that feels less grinding on a constant basis, urges reduce and compulsivity dilutes.

The four elements: air, earth, water and fire

Elan Shapiro (2012) framed emotional regulation into "*The Four Elements*". I like it because it is easy for clients to remember.

Air: breathing
Earth: grounding
Water: salivating
Fire: visualisation

Air: breathing

Breathing mindfully is usually one of the first methods for stress-busting and emotional regulation. We therapists can teach our clients our favourite mindful breathing, such as diaphragmatic breathing or *Ujjayi* (ocean) breathing (Marich, 2014, pp. 140–1). Clients can find their own as well. You can ask clients to practice different types of breathing and to encourage them to be mindful of how they breathe. The main aim with breathing exercises is to breathe out for longer than breathing in, as this allows the body to absorb oxygen effectively and soothes the nervous system.

Earth: grounding

When we encounter difficult memories or emotions, it is important to feel the floor underneath our feet. We can lose touch of our own sense of our body when we are overwhelmed. I ask my clients to pay attention to their feet. They can move their feet from toes to heal and from side to side to have a better awareness of how they make contact with the floor. If they are in an high state of emotion, for example, they had a difficult conflict with their partner just before coming to their session, I would ask them to stand and breathe and rock gently on their feet from side to side and back and forth, gently, just enough to notice the weight of their body on their leg and feet. This is usually a calming and soothing process.

Water: salivating

It is a less known regulation method yet an efficient and easy one. The sympathetic nervous system is activated in moments of distress. When a person feels acute anxiety, fear or anger, the mouth will become dry. By self-salivating, we can re-engage the parasympathetic nervous system and calm down our emotions. Some clients can find it difficult to self-salivate on their own, but they can help themselves with sipping water or sucking on a sweet or mint.

Fire: visualisation

This is the same principles of an internal safe place discussed above. However, you can also encourage the client to have other images to call up in their mind that can help with emotional regulation. It may be a mental snapshot of a loved one, or a pet, a beautiful place, or a favourite colour. Psychotherapists can invite the client into guided visualisations for urge reduction too. I use different ones depending on the client. One that I often use sounds like this:

> An urge comes and goes, always comes and goes, just like the waves of an ocean. Imagine standing bare feet on the wet sand of a beach, by the ocean. The wave comes and envelopes your feet with water, the sand covers your feet. You don't need to do anything, just breathe and observe, because you know pretty soon the wave will go, the water will withdraw, the sand will be taken with the water, and you can see your feet again. Back and forth. If you wait long enough, just a minute or two, the urge will naturally go. There is nothing you need to do, just wait and observe.

Another helpful visualisation is what I call the Parent-Child conversation:

> Imagine there's the most delicious chocolate cake in front of you. You want to it eat all, and you want to eat it now. Your mouth is salivating and your heart is racing at the anticipation of pleasure eating that cake. Imagine that the wise and nurturing parent part of you comes and hugs you and says: 'I know you want to eat the whole chocolate cake now. It is so tempting, isn't it? But you can wait. You can wait. You can have a scrumptious piece later. Only one delicious piece later. But not now. Just wait a little longer and attend to your other needs now. The chocolate cake will still be here later, I promise.

Mind flexibility

Flexibility in the early stages of therapy can be helpful for the longer-term success of treatment. This can be introduced as a form of a light challenge. I usually propose the following to my clients:

> We all do some things the same way, in the same order because we are humans, and we are creatures of habits. Compulsivity is not the same from having habits, of course, but it does sit in a system that is stuck. One way to loosen up the system is to challenge yourself in doing some small things differently. Slowly, your mind will be more used to flexibility. What could be some small things that you always do the same way that you could do differently, just once, just to try what it feels like?

Some clients respond with:

> I'm going to wear odd socks at work.
> I always have breakfast before having a shower. Tomorrow I will have a shower before breakfast.

Clients are usually surprised that even those small little changes can bring low level anxiety, but they also learn that they can survive changes.

There are benefits to mind flexibility. It helps with problem solving by seeing things from different points of view and it creates a greater sense of self-efficacy. Psychologist Albert Bandura (1997) teaches us that self-efficacy is an important factor for well-being. He asserts that people with self-efficacy are healthier and more successful than those with low self-efficacy expectations.

The more clients find mind flexibility difficult, the more blocks there will be in therapy, and therefore the more patient and slow we will have to be, paying particular attention to building the therapeutic alliance (Muran and Barber, 2010).

Emotional regulation for shame reduction

One of the central maintaining factors of sexual compulsivity is shame. In Part 1 of this book, I stressed the importance of clinicians equipping themselves with the up to date sexology knowledge to avoid accidental 'conversion therapy'. It is the linking of sexual experiences to a moral code that elicits self-shame, resulting in people judging themselves as bad and wrong rather than different and still ok. The normalisation of their legal and consensual sexual behaviours, feelings, fantasies and experiences is crucial to shame reduction; it will disrupt the moebius loop of shame.

It is also important to remind clients that shame tries to say: '*you're wrong*', it is when there is a toxic fusion between what we do and who we are. Brené Brown defines shame as:

> the intense painful feeling or experience of believing we are flawed and therefore unworthy of love and belonging (2012, p. 69).

Shame operates at a survival level, effectively stopping us from doing something to exclude us from the safety of our social group. In this way, the level of shame that we feel is a metric of how much we care, not how bad we are. We feel shame because we care deeply about social connection and shared codes of behaviour. People who are 'shameless' have no empathy or concern for others. The positive function of shame is that it forces withdrawal and time to reflect on behaviour whilst alerting us to our deepest need to connect. Unfortunately, internal shame dialogue gets internalised into worthlessness and encourages behaviours to defend against the pain of shame, like sexual behaviours.

Shame reduction and resilience is learning the skills to separate what we do from who we are. Brown describes beautifully what shame resilience is like:

> You still want folks to like respect, and even admire what you've created, but your self-worth is not on the table. You know that you are far more than a painting, an innovative idea, an effective pitch, a good sermon, or a high Amazon.com ranking. Yes, it will be disappointing and difficult if your friends or colleagues don't share your enthusiasm, or if things don't go well, but this effort is about what you do, not who you are. Regardless of the outcome, you've already dared greatly, and that's totally aligned with your values; with who you want to be (2012, p. 64).

The antidote to shame is empathy and shame is healed in relationship (Brown, 2012). The therapy space is a precious space of full acceptance, regardless of clients' behaviours, experiences and practises, so long as they are legal and consensual. Working with shame requires careful pacing. If we respond to clients' shame with an immediate reaction of kindness, clients will feel our urgency and shame will increase. First, therapists need to hold the shame for clients, be there with them in their difficult experiences of shame, and then slowly guiding them to face it.

Dayton (2000) outlines four steps in assisting shame-based clients to unravel feelings:

1   Feel the fullness of the emotion
2   Label it
3   Explore its meaning and function within the self
4   Choose whether or not to communicate the inner state with another person

I often see clients' shame speaking through their body posture. Their bodies look like they're sinking into the couch, their head collapsing on their shoulders, almost as though they want to disappear. Body posture locks emotion in preventing us from accessing another emotional state (Veenstra et al., 2016). We can reduce shame by asking clients to make voluntary movements that is counter-shame. For example, I ask clients to stand up, move around, look up, look at me, raise their hands to the ceiling with fingers wide, and I ask them to make sure they have a straight back. Sometimes I suggest the homework of paying attention to how they walk in the streets, making their body feel tall.

Another way to address shame with clients is to make them aware of the different parts of themselves. Ask the client to identify the characteristics of their inner critic, the part that shames them. Ask them whose voice the critic speaks with. Is it theirs, or one of their parents'? Encourage them to give this part a full physical description and name, 'Critical Pete' 'Raging Sally' 'Mr Angry Pants'. Don't be afraid to use humour. Elicit the good intentions of the critic. Is it trying to keep the client safe, help them to do well, keep them out of trouble? Ask the critic part how old it thinks the client is. It is likely to think the client is very young. Externalise the shame voice so that the client can objectify it rather than identify with it. The next step is to encourage the client to invite another part of themselves into the conversation. It may be the 'Wisdom Part', or 'My Adult Self'. Ask this wise part to correct the shaming part. For example: 'I'm a terrible cook' Vs 'I manage to make a nutritional meal the best way I can'.

Paul Gilbert offers rich ideas of self-compassion in his book "*The Compassionate Mind*" (2013). He writes about "*compassionate self-correction*" to counter-act "*Shame-based self-attacking*". Some of these are: focusing on the desire to improve, emphasising growth, being forward-looking and building on the positive (2013, p. 373). Gilbert proposes that some of the compassionate attributes are:

> motivation to be more caring of self and others" and "the ability to tolerate rather than avoid difficult feelings, memories or situations (2013, p. 236).

In practical terms, self-compassion to reduce shame looks something like that:

1 *I feel bad about myself.*
2 *My feeling bad is my shame.*
3 *I'm going to take a moment and breathe through this feeling.*
4 *I'm feeling the shame and I accept myself too.*
5 *Even though I feel shame I can love myself.* Client can put a warm hand on the part of the body that is soothing, the Heart Centre for example, saying gently. *I am a human being worthy of love.*
6 *Everybody feels bad sometimes. It is a human experience to have unpleasant feelings.*

This is only meant to be a guide, the process will be slightly different, depending on clients and the situations.

Emotional regulation for managing the partner's upset

The impact of witnessing their partner's pain will be intense and have affects turned either inwards and outwards, or both. Some common inwards affects are increased shame, self-loathing, anger at themselves, despair, depression and self-harm. Some outwards affects are anger at the partner, anger at childhood, anger at the world, projection and blaming their partner, over-working, checking out, being impatient and irritated with their partner wanting them to 'get over it' quickly.

For clinicians, it is a delicate balance to allocate enough space in our consultations for helping our clients manage the upheavals at home in their here-and-now as well as the thorough exploration of their Erotic Template.

There are three elements to consider when helping clients manage their emotions with their partner's upset: emotional regulation, communication skills and psycho-education on do's and don't's.

Emotional regulation

All the emotional regulations described above will be useful for the client when managing their feelings about their partners. The more emotional regulation techniques clients have the better. If the partner is willing, some of the emotional regulation methods can be done together, for example, they can learn to breathe mindfully together.

Communication skills

Rosenberg (2015) explains that non-violent communication is a process by which people can express honestly and receive empathically through the following four components:

1   Observations: the concrete actions we observe that affect our well-being
2   Feelings: how we feel in relation to what we observe
3   Needs: the needs, values, desires that create our feelings
4   Requests: the concrete actions we request in order to enrich our lives
    (2015, p. 7).

Here is an example from someone who wants to speak to their betrayed partner: '*I see tears in your eyes. I feel remorse because I know I hurt you which is against my values and desires. I would like us to be kind to each other when we are hurt*'.

Helping clients with better communication with their partner means that they can regulate some of the relational tension or bad atmosphere in the household, which can be ongoing for some couples. My golden rules to help with starting to repair the chaos of the betrayal are:

1   Having a language of accountability: '*I do as I say*'.
2   Having a language of responsibility: '*I know I have done this to you*'.
3   Being proactive: go towards partner and ask them what they need if clients notice they're upset.
4   Starting sentences with '*I*' instead of '*you*' to avoid sounding critical.

5   Remain self-compassionate and compassionate to their partner. Partners won't heal quickly, the mistrust will linger for a long time. Clients have to remain with compassion not to force their partner to '*get better*' soon.

6   Stay empathic. Clients need to stay mindful about what it must be like for their partner. Their world is turned upside down. Their relationship is no longer reality for them. Sexual information that clients have known for a long time is all new to their partner. They will need time to digest it all. Be patient, give the partner plenty of time and space when they need it.

7   Take breaks. It's ok to go in separate rooms when things are too tough. Go out for a bit to diffuse anger and other emotions.

8   Don't overshare information of a sexual nature – it may become a trigger to the partner. It may relieve our clients of their guilt but it may be a burden for their partner to carry.

Domestic abuse and violence

The discovery of sexual compulsivity can produce intense emotions greater than is tolerable for some people. Some may resort to psychological or physical violence. Partners who have been betrayed could become abusive. We therapists are well-attuned to identify signs of domestic abuse when it is a man doing it to a woman, for good reasons, as the statistics show the prevalence of this abuse to women. Men are typically physically stronger and can cause a lot more damage to women than the other way around. In many cases of CSB, it is the woman who is betrayed by their male partner, and the female partner can then be the one to lash out. Psychotherapists must not fall into a gender bias and minimise physical or psychological abuse by a woman towards a man or by a same-sex partners of equal strength. I have seen many women thinking it was ok to slap their husbands or throw things at them after the discovery of betrayal. Some also think it is ok to be repeatedly verbally abusive. Men on the receiving end do not often think the violence is unacceptable because their shame tells them they deserve it.

Equally, some of the behaviours that someone with CSB can do to keep hiding their secret sexual behaviours may fall under the domestic abuse and violence definition. The UK Government published the following statement on Intimate Partner Violence (IPV):

The cross-government definition of domestic violence and abuse is any incident or pattern of incidents of controlling, coercive, threatening behaviour, violence or abuse between those aged 16 or over who are, or have been, intimate partners or family members regardless of gender or sexuality. The abuse can encompass, but is not limited to:

- psychological
- physical
- sexual
- financial
- emotional.

These may present in various ways. For example:

1 Sharing sexually explicit images of a partner. People with CSB may share an explicit image of their partner to a secret lover without their partner's consent. If a betrayed partner finds some videos of their spouse engaging in sexual activities with another, sharing these without their partner's consent is also abusive.
2 Restricting access to money. After the discovery of a betrayal, especially one that involved a large amount of money, the betrayed partner may decide to control the money of the betrayer.
3 Repeated put downs. It is not uncommon for a betrayed person to continuously put down a betrayer after discovery. Also, many betrayers can repeatedly put down their betrayed partner by telling them they're not good enough.
4 Preventing a partner from seeing family/friends. On some occasions, the betrayed partner will find out that the betrayer engaged in sexual compulsivity with the help of a friend who, perhaps, encouraged getting drunk and visits to strip clubs. The betrayed may force the betrayer not to see this kind of people again.
5 Threats, harassments and creating fear. The betrayer may use threats to keep the betrayed compliant so that they can continue their non-consensual non-monogamy behaviours. For example, they may threaten their partner with aggression and tell them '*you make me do this*'. Equally, the betrayed can use threats to keep the betrayer on the '*straight and narrow*'. For example, some betrayed people will threaten the betrayer that they will divulge some of their sexual behaviours to their boss or parents if they don't do as they say.
6 Tracking devices. It is unacceptable to monitor a person using online communication tools or spyware, however some betrayed partners may coerce the betrayer into doing so or they may install a device without their partner's consent.
7 Extreme jealousy. It is a normal reaction of betrayal to be jealous, but extreme jealousy is when the betrayed is so consumed by it that they attempt to control their partner using threats or humiliation. Equally, someone with CSB may also be extremely jealous if their partner decides they want to meet other people too and may want to use unacceptable control.
8 Forcing a partner to obey their rules. A betrayed partner may impose a no pornography and no masturbation rule for their partner against their

consent and a threat of divorce if they breach that rule. Equally, someone with CSB can impose rules on their partners such as '*if you give me a blowjob every day I won't cheat*'.

9   Controlling clothing. Someone with CSB may force their partner to wear certain types of clothing to turn them on despite their partner saying they don't like it. If someone with CSB doesn't own their erotic, they might force their partner not to show any parts of their body as they believe their partner's sexuality is the cause of their sexual problems.

10 Forcing to do things they don't want to. This includes behaviours often seen from a betrayer to a betrayed before the discovery of sexual compulsivity, for example forcing a partner to have sex when they don't want to, or forcing them to look at pornographic material or have sex with others when they don't want to.

It is rare for clients and their partner to recognise, acknowledge and name domestic abuse when there is so much to process after the discovery of sexual compulsivity. Psychotherapists have to remain alert and address these behaviours without any gender bias when they are presented.

References

Bandura, A. (1997). *Self-efficacy: the exercise of control.* New York: Worth.

Brown, B. (2012). *Daring greatly: how the courage to be vulnerable transforms the way we live, love, parent and lead.* London: Portfolio Penguin.

Dayton, T. (2000). *Trauma and addiction: ending the cycle of pain through emotional literacy.* Deerfield Beach, FL, USA: Health Communications.

Gilbert, P. (2013). *The compassionate mind.* London: Robinson.

Marich, J. (2014). *Trauma made simple.* Eau Claire, WI: PESI Publishing and Media.

Muran, J.C. and Barber J.P. (2010). *The therapeutic alliance.* New York: Guilford Press.

Rosenberg, M.B. (2015). *Nonviolent communication: a language of life.* Encinitas, CA: PuddleDancer Press.

Shapiro, E. (2012). 4 elements exercises for stress reduction. [Available Online]: http://emdrresearchfoundation.org/toolkit/four-elements.pdf.

UK Government website on IPV. [Available online]: https://www.gov.uk/guidance/intimate-partner-violence-domestic-abuse-programmes.

Veenstra et al. (2016). Embodied mood regulation: the impact of body posture on mood recovery, negative thoughts, and mood-congruent recall. *Cognition Emotion*, 31(7), 1361–76.

Wells, A. (2009). *Metacognitive therapy for anxiety and depression.* New York: The Guildford Press.

Chapter 11

Phase 2: Reprocessing

Treating compulsivity

When clients have enough impulse control, emotional regulation for urge reduction and shame reduction, psychotherapists can guide the treatment towards the underlying causes of the compulsive sexual behaviours. As discussed in Part 2 of this book, the underlying causes of compulsivity are varied: unresolved trauma, attachment difficulties, poor self-esteem, narcissistic traits, high sexual desire and unresolved psychosexual problems. In my experience, the recovery from all of these disturbances is connection.

Being connection-focused

The main goal of the reprocessing phase is to look at the client's entire life story so that they can understand fully how they got to where they are, without judgements, without blaming, but with a thorough understanding of their processes and patterns in terms of emotions, behaviours, core beliefs, attachment styles, and so on. Depending on what was identified as predisposing and precipitating factors of their sexual compulsivity, the reprocessing might take different shapes of treatment.

Within the pluralistic framework, therapists can treat a client's compulsive sexual behaviours by being connection-focused, because we humans are connection-focused creatures. Through the lens of connection we can help the client understand their life, interweaving all the facets of their selves. Therapists can do so whilst remaining faithful to their own existing modalities, whether it is person-centred, behavioural, psychodynamic, or integrative, although it does help to be humanistic and relational. Psychotherapists can guide clients into understanding their various connections:

Connection with self. Their sense of self-worth, self-esteem, self-efficacy. Their internal conscious and unconscious script about themselves. Their sense of their sexuality and their gender.

Connection with meaningful others. How they express and receive love and care to and from others. The internal conscious and unconscious scripts they have about relationships.

Connection with non-meaningful others. How they assign unconscious roles to others who are not part of their intimate circles, for example, roles of father, mother, rulers, aggressors, carers. These roles are typically assigned unconsciously onto colleagues, managers, sex workers, wider family, acquaintances.

Connection with the world. Their sense of standing in the world and taking their rightful space unapologetically. Their internal conscious and unconscious script about society and the world. For some people the world can be persecutory, for others it may be perceived as unrealistically fair. Connection with the world may include paying attention to their connection with nature, which is also meaningful and healing for many people.

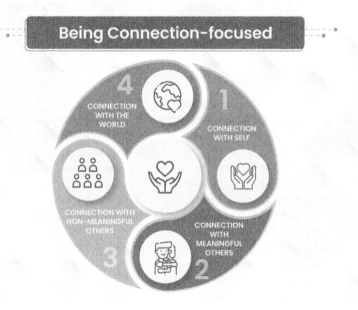

With the connection-focused approach in mind every conversation about CSB may be of therapeutic use when linking the conversations to their different connections.

Jacob loves having long sexual events because he enjoys the feeling of being exuberant in his erotic (connection with self). His partner criticises him for it because she prefers neat and tidy sex that doesn't take long. He feels hurt for being misunderstood by his partner (connection with meaningful other), the hurt goes deep because it reminds him of his critical mother who didn't like when he was an exuberant child (connection with meaningful other). To soothe his hurt he fantasises about seeing a sex worker who will understand him better (connection with non-meaningful other). He doesn't feel he can talk to his wife about it because he believes the world is unkind and his needs won't be met unless he pays someone to do so (connection to the world).

In my work, I find that bringing connection to the client's awareness on a regular basis helps them to be seen fully by us and act as a healing agent. As babies, we only have the eyes of our primary care givers to help us understand who we are. Then, we have our peers, and intimate relationships. When the psychotherapeutic relationship is strong, it is a potent source of connection where clients can re-evaluate themselves and change how they see their core selves through the nurturing, non-judgmental and unconditional positive regard of their therapist.

Phase 2 helps clients with owning their own story to reduce projection of their dis-owned parts onto others. Therapists can encourage their clients honest appraisal of their childhood, loss and grief, their sexual anxieties and their low self-esteem, which includes the commitment of self-care to themselves.

Working with trauma

Phase 2 often requires reprocessing significant trauma and intense grief. Psychotherapists must be confident that clients have enough Phase 1 emotional resources to enter this part of the therapy to ensure safe trauma treatment (Rothschild, 2010). When engaging in trauma psychotherapy work it is important to make sure that all these sessions are framed with emotional regulation and grounding at the beginning and the end of each session for safe practice. I keep a tight structure for my trauma-oriented sessions. My 50-minute trauma reprocessing sessions are structured like this:

10 minutes: arriving, checking in and anchoring in safe place.
30 minutes: trauma processing (Somatic trauma therapy, Chairwork, EMDR or other trauma interventions)
10 minutes: anchoring in safe place. A brief meaning making conversation. Self-care discussion.

Trauma psychotherapy involves working with the body, the nervous system as well as our brain and cognitions (Rothschild, 2017). Connectedness is a biological process felt in our body, which helps regulate our nervous system through the vagus nerve (Porges and Dana, 2018). We self-regulate through co-regulation; mammals co-regulate through social engagement and social bonding. We achieve attunement through eye contact and touch. Our level of availability for here-and-now connection will depend on our physiology, whether we are tired, hungry, anxious, upset or rested, relaxed and content. The absence of threat in itself isn't enough to make us feel safe, we also need safe social engagement and bonding. Relational psychotherapy offers that: a consistent, reliable, predictable therapeutic relationship with the client.

Some of the tried and tested methods of trauma therapy are:

1 **Butterfly hugs.** Gently tap just below the collar bone, right and left, in slow or quick successions, whilst breathing gently. Clients can do this whilst thinking of a positive thought about themselves.
2 **Tense and release.** Clients can tense all their muscles up tight, then slowly release.
3 **Mindfulness through sensory soothers.** Ask clients to use items that can soothe their senses, such as soft fabrics, essential oils, teddy bear, calming music. Ask clients to turn their attention to the sensation of touching or smelling these items, leaving the trauma memories behind for now. This teaches clients the skill of mindfully attending to the present, whilst giving the client a pleasurable, soothing, sensory experience. This exercise is also helpful because it creates new positive somatic markers.
4 **Adrenaline releasers.** When we are in a threat response, our bodies fill up with adrenaline and cortisol to prepare for fight or flight. At that moment, sitting still may not be a good solution because the energy has nowhere to go. We need to move our bodies vigorously: running up and down stairs, doing star jumps, going for a walk or a run, punching a cushion, marching around the room, dancing to loud music. These activities release the stress hormones and calm the body and the mind. In the consulting room, there will be limitations as to what clients can do, but these are good suggestions for clients to try in between sessions.
5 **Writing.** Some clients find writing about the trauma experience easier than speaking about it. There is no right or wrong in doing so. They can write in scribbles, or drawings, then rip it up or throw away. It could be written as a story, in which the client is the main character or the narrator. An important step could be to invite the client to rewrite the ending. Some clients can write their stories into fiction or poems. One of my clients turned their traumatic stories into songs, which they recorded. We listened to them together. It was a wonderful healing moment. This experience can be cathartic for some clients.
6 **Visualising and re-enacting the trauma story.** Sometimes, clients need to enact what they wished they could have done at the time, either with visual imagination or body movements (Levine, 1997; Rothschild, 2017). Ask the client to visualise and replay the event introducing the things they wished could have happened, like beating off their attacker or running away from the scene. In the therapy room, invite the client to physically enact running away, (pumping their hands and feet whilst remaining seated) or punching the abuser, (using a cushion) or shouting for help. These interventions can release the trauma from both the mind (visualisation) and body (physical re-enactment).

7   **Changing the sensory qualities of the trauma experience.** Some traumatic memories are embedded somatic markers of our five senses: visual, auditory, touch, olfactory and taste. We can take the emotional charge out of a specific trauma by guiding the client to change the sensory qualities of the memory. They can indicate whether the client is associated or dissociated from the traumatic event. Deliberately moving between association and dissociation can reduce the power of the memory. For example, you can ask a client to take a photograph of their traumatic memory in their mind's eye, so that the image is static rather than moving. Then, ask clients to turn the photograph into black or white, or change some colours. Sometimes, you might ask a client to put something else in the photograph that is incongruent with the trauma or even ridiculous (one client chose to have the people in the photograph in Santa Clause outfits). Some clients may want to imagine that photograph being framed and moving away from them, others prefer to imagine they shred the photograph. You can do the same process with the other senses. One client had the intrusive taste of their abuser's penis in his mouth. By imagining a different taste, some of the traumatic charge was released.

For clients whose sexual behaviour problems are caused by high sexual desire, Phase 2 is mostly a time to work towards full acceptance of their sexual desire level and how to align it to their relationships, values and their meaningful connections. If this is done with shame-reducing normalisation and sex-positivity, Phase 2 may be brief for these clients.

For clients who identified an unresolved psychosexual problem as a predisposing or precipitating factor of their CSB, classic sex therapy methods may be appropriate for Phase 2. Sensate Focus is one of the main sex therapy interventions, however it is important to assess the relationship before recommending it. If the partner is hurt by the discovery of CSB, it won't be appropriate to recommend Sensate Focus for the couple until the partner is ready, but in the meantime, self-sensate focus can be done. Other sex therapy interventions can be very useful too such as 'stop-start (for rapid ejaculation), 'waxing and waning' (erectile problems), 'mindful masturbation' (delayed ejaculation), Kegel exercises for various sexual problems including vaginismus (Kaplan, 1974–1989; Hawton, 1985; Laffy, 2013).

Therapists can spend a good amount of time in Phase 2 helping clients unpack their life with a connection-focused and relational approach. This will help treat the underlying disturbances such as poor self-esteem and attachment problems. I want to acknowledge that an important part of the CSB treatment using my model relies on the psychotherapists' common sense and their clinical intuition. I do not believe in formulaic approaches that take away the therapists' creativity.

References

Hawton, K. (1985). *Sex therapy: a practical guide*. New York: Oxford University Press.

Kaplan, H.S. (1974). *The new sex therapy*. New York: Brunner/Mazel.

Kaplan, H.S. (1989). *PE: how to overcome premature ejaculation*. Abingdon: Taylor and Francis Group.

Laffy, C. (2013). *LoveSex: an integrative model for sexual education*. London: Karnac Books.

Levine, P.A. (1997). *Waking the tiger: healing trauma*. Berkeley, CA: North Atlantic Books.

Porges, S.W. and Dana, D. (2018). *Clinical applications of the polyvagal theory: the emergence of polyvagal-informed therapies*. New York: W.W. Norton & Company.

Rothschild, B. (2010). *8 keys to safe trauma recovery*. New York: W.W. Norton & Company.

Rothschild, B. (2017). *The body remembers, volume 2. Revolutionizing trauma treatment*. New York: W.W. Norton & Company.

Sale, J. (2020). CICS: working with trauma and shame. *Contemporary Institute of Clinical Sexology*.

Chapter 12

Phase 3: Reconstruction

Meaning making

The last phase focuses on the existential process of clients, integrating all the meaning-making discoveries they made through healing, and re-adjusting to a new sense of their selves. For example core beliefs such as '*I'm helpless*' can transform into '*I have control over my choices*'. Phase 3 aims to integrate those more helpful core beliefs into a new system that clients create for themselves, hence getting their full, delicious pie of life. Their commitment to self-care is a permanent change because it comes from the clients' own understanding of their core selves. The ultimate goal is for clients to be in full awareness of their here-and-now and how to be resilient to life adversities so that they can manage difficult times with many different resources.

Phase 3 also looks at maintaining a thriving sex life free of shame in line with the WAS declaration of sexual pleasure mentioned in Part 1. Psychotherapists can help clients have a clear vision of the future, knowing what they want for themselves and how to achieve it. It is important to keep in mind that Phase 3 is not about figuring out a life plan that is rigid and unchanging. It is often the rigid rules and unchanging commitments that maintain CSB, so we don't want to recreate that. Maintenance of a good life is the opposite. It is about psychological and emotional flexibility and having the courage to re-evaluate commitments on a regular basis. The one certainty is that life does change and we change as we age, we create new meaning with new life experiences, our sense of connection with ourselves, others and the world over time. When my clients are in a place of well-being at the end of their treatment and they are making their commitment to self-care, I encourage them to keep reviewing these commitments, once a year at least. If they managed to repair their relationship, I also encourage that they review the couple's commitment on a regular basis. Nothing about being human is ever set in stone. Once again, I often use the analogy of food. I say something like:

> On a rainy day, I sometimes want chips because it's warming and comforting. But it doesn't mean I will always want chips on a rainy day. Sometimes I might want a pizza. On sunny days I might sometimes want

an ice cream, but other times I'd crave a tomato salad. All we need to do for our well-being is being super aware of our emotional needs so that we can be conscious about what is going on for us, rather than ending up stuffing ourselves with chips not knowing why. As we become conscious and aware, we can also express to our partner what is going on for us so that they know how to navigate the relational space. If they assume that you'd want chips on every rainy day, they might get surprised when you suddenly show up with a pizza!.

This makes for a light conversation, but clients usually understand this very well when explained in that way.

Kinsukuroi

When a vase is broken we want to glue it back together and pretend it had never been broken. Does it ever work? We can somehow always see the cracks we're trying to hide. Although sexual compulsivity is not desirable, it may be the very struggle that gets people to face the hidden cracks of their childhood as well as the ones they made in their adult lives. Therapy is hard, but it is a great opportunity to heal properly. Healing is not only about putting the broken vase back together, but it is to get the gold in the cracks. A Japanese pottery art called '*Kintsugi*' (golden joinery) or, more appropriately in the context of therapy, '*Kinsukuroi*' (golden repair), doesn't hide the cracks of their pottery, instead it enhances them by joining the pieces together with gold. I often show a picture of '*Kinsukuroi*' to my clients to explain to them what the end of therapy looks like. I think it is a great image to represent what psychological integration looks like. I would quite like to rename therapy 'golden repair'.

Frankl (2004) gives us his accounts on surviving the Holocaust in his powerful thought-provoking book *Man's Search For Meaning* and his observation of the human existence being capable of great love and hatred; the humankind capacity to lean towards the beauty and the ugliness. Frankl experienced being robbed of all of his identities and statuses. What is left of our sense of being human when all that we associate with is gone? Surviving trauma and grief changes us, it enhances our sense of self, it gives us a new perspective on the joy of living and thriving.

References

Frankl, V.E. (2004). *Man's search for meaning*. London: Rider, Random House Group.
World Association for Sexual Health (WAS): Declaration of sexual pleasure. [Available online]: https://worldsexualhealth.net/declaration-on-sexual-pleasure/.

Chapter 13

Clients stories

Treatment

Heterosexual men

Roger

One of the most useful ideas for Roger was a soothing object which helped with his impulse control. He bought a pendant with his birthstone that he could wear around his neck and touch in moments of stress. The birthstone was meaningful for him because he had been unwanted by his mother at birth. Muscle toning worked well for him too as it was something easy he could integrate in his everyday life. When he took time for his passionate engagement, he was apologetic about it to Megan. I challenged him. He had quite a lot to apologise for; but starting a hobby wasn't it. Owning for himself the things that were not an apology was essential as it connected to his childhood where he felt he had to apologise for his very existence (connection with self, others and the world).

Roger's unrelenting work schedule was one of the maintaining factors of CSB and it was part of his moebius loop of shame which became a chronic stress. He didn't feel he could speak to Megan about his emotional diffi- culties because he already felt like a bad husband and feared she would leave him if he wasn't perfect due to his anxious attachment style. He self-soothed with other people instead. Roger needed to loosen his tight loop of shame. Roger's connection with self was built through the eyes of his unloving, rejecting mother. It made perfect sense that his core belief would be '*I'm worthless*', which brought up much pain. To soothe it, Roger chose the strategy to dis-own his vulnerability; he thought that reaching for perfection would be the good antidote to '*I'm worthless*'; but he realised in therapy that it was the wrong one. The antidote to '*I'm worthless*' actually was '*I'm worthy*'. That was unchartered territory for him. Being touched and seen without any fear of rejection was crucial for him and he thought it could only be done by someone he paid, because he mistrusted other people, in- cluding Megan. He did not assimilate that Megan loved him without jud- gements. With CBT questioning (Greenberger and Padesky, 1995), I asked

Roger to look for the evidence that reinforced the thoughts '*Megan is like my parents*'. There weren't any. Even now, after the discovery of his CSB, Megan was still loving!

I introduced the concept of '*Ego States*' in the language of Transactional Analysis (Berne, 2009) to continue the discussion on how he could understand the projection of his childhood onto his here-and-now. When he was in his Adult Ego State he could brainstorm, express his emotions, ask for help, deliberate new ways of doing things. I asked Roger to use his dual awareness, noticing the somatic and emotional difference when he was in his Child Ego State and Adult Ego State, back and forth so that it could be easier to identifying them when they got activated. This brought major changes in his everyday life because he became aware when he was feeling a fear of rejection at work, or feeling abandoned by Megan. He was able to understand on an emotional level that sex workers were the rescuers to his Inner Child.

Session after session, Roger could no longer ignore all the pain of his childhood. The Chairwork intervention is a powerful trauma treatment (Kellogg, 2015). I asked Roger to write a letter to his mother, not to send it but to bring it to therapy. I suggested that he did so in small steps, for a short time, as it could be an intense experience and I wanted to avoid overwhelming him. In session, I encouraged Roger to read the letter expressing the raw parts of his wounds with Chairwork, imagining his mother sat in one of the chairs, whilst feeling safe in my consulting room. Much anger and pain came up, but he felt some healing happening. We did the same process with his father and finally his brother, who was the most difficult one to process. The last Chairwork session was with his Inner Child, speaking to his younger self sending him love. This was probably the most reparative session for him. Through the Chairwork experience, a new narrative emerged for Roger; he was strong to survive his childhood. He did hurt Megan and himself but he also built a good home and had two balanced teenagers. He changed from being a '*people-pleaser*' to expressing his boundaries at work and at home. He could then connect emotionally with new core beliefs '*I'm worthy to be me*', '*I'm worthy to exist*', '*I'm worthy to have my own space*', '*I'm worthy to be loved*'. Megan, who was courageous enough to have her own therapy after the discovery, noticed stark changes in Roger and decided to stay in the marriage.

By the time he began Phase 3, Roger reported feeling in control of his sexual behaviours with no more compulsion; he was fully aware of his emotional and cognitive processes. At the end of therapy, Roger described having the best sex life he had ever had with Megan and he had a new existential understanding of himself; although he was not loved as a child, it wasn't because of his defectiveness but because of the inability of his family of origin to love him.

Martin

I normalised Martin's use of pornography and masturbation as a *'good strategy'* for emotional regulation, which worked well for him as a teenager when he was faced with the enormous pain of his mother passing away; but now it was time to add more strategies alongside pornography and masturbation. He particularly liked mindfulness as emotional regulation; he downloaded an app and took his practice further. As he developed other ways to manage stress, anger and boredom, he reported that his pornography and masturbation strategy was no longer centre stage.

Fairburn (2013) proposes the use of alternative activities to reduce urges in the context of binge eating. I found it useful with impulse control to surf sexual urges. Fairburn asserts that the alternative activities need to have three properties: (1) active, (2) enjoyable and (3) realistic. Martin chose swimming, which he enjoyed and set him up for a productive day. In times of urges, he chose his alternative activity of watching Netflix documentaries that he was interested in. It is an active action because it is watching something of interest, so there is an intellectual engagement, rather than watching a screen passively. By doing these activities, he increased his sense of self-efficacy, which raised his self-esteem.

We identified that Martin needed to engage in psychosexual therapy and learn how to masturbate mindfully with a gentler hand grip; being aware of all the sensations. It served as cognitive re-framing to think about masturbation not being about escaping something but about pleasurable high-quality time of solo sex. I suggested he used organic lube to send a psychological message: *'your sex life deserves the best'*.

The second part of his psychosexual intervention was to help Martin speak honestly about sex with Amy. It turned out that Amy really liked having those conversations and she was relieved to see him keen to be sexual with her as she was starting to lose hope that he was interested. He gained information about what she liked sexually that he had not known before. Sexual excitement increased between them.

I invited Martin to process his mother's death. First, we discussed some of the good memories that he had of his mother. We did a visualisation exercise of him remembering her hugs and the house where he grew up. He was then able to start talking about what he remembered when she died. He got in touch with rage and loneliness. Together we were able to identify two incorrect central narrative he made up as a child: *'my mother left me because she didn't love him'*; and *'my father stopped loving me because I caused her death'*. Connecting with these childhood stories, he rationalised them in the here-and-now; those stories couldn't be true. Instead, we discussed the true story, a more unsettling one: there were no reasons for the untimely death of his mother; it happened out of bad luck. Although more unsettling, it was based on a solid existential truth that became a relief for Martin. Together, we discussed all the events of his life that his mother couldn't witness: growing up, meeting Amy, getting his qualifications, being the 25-year-old man that he now was. I became the witness of his life, a therapeutic connection within which he could grieve. Martin learnt that it was ok to feel sadness when thinking about his mother; the loss will always be there. Now that he knew how to meet his emotional world, he didn't need to desensitise himself with pornography. Compulsion disappeared. He now watched pornography and masturbated when he had the time, with clear time boundaries so that other areas of his life weren't affected. His pornography and masturbation time was his 'solo good quality sex time' and sometimes it was his 'stress relief time', without any shame. Amy knew about it and she was happy with it because their sex life had improved with more open and honest conversation. Martin described himself as 'grown up'; being in an adult place he could share with Amy, whilst meeting the six principles of sexual health.

When Martin felt the time was right, he decided to do another 'funeral' ritual for his mother on her death anniversary because he didn't remember her actual funeral. He chose to do it in session with me. He brought a picture of her, we dimmed the lights, he played her favourite music, he made a speech about her and he said goodbye to her, witnessed by me. It was a meaningful moment of great connection.

Women

Francesca

Francesca's position '*I'm OK – You're not OK*' showed up in the therapeutic relationship by calling therapists '*charlatans*'. It seemed she spent a lot of time reading stories of therapists breaching their ethics and sleeping with their patients. I asked her if she was wondering how strong my ethical boundaries were. Seducing men into falling in lust with her was one of her ways of operating in the world. Was she trying the same operating method with me? She consistently arrived late at her appointments, asked me if I could extend the session to make up for her 50 minutes. I refused. She would be angry at my refusal. Occasionally she would not turn up, when I charged her for the missed sessions, she would get angry. I asked her what she had hoped would happen. Did she want to be so special that my boundaries wouldn't matter? Did she hope our signed agreement would be overlooked?

I helped her see that feeling special at the expense of boundaries was the same theme as her sexual abuse story. My refusal to ignore my boundaries was not a rejection of her but a refusal to repeat the story of her childhood. When she could see, for the first time in her life, that boundaries were caring and loving, she changed, she became more settled in therapy. Establishing our therapeutic relationship was a long process. It took over six months for

Francesca to commit to therapy and turning up on time with no more cancellations. It took another six months for her to learn and practice some good emotional regulations for her self-care and impulse control.

The sexual trauma that Francesca endured breached her sexual and relational integrity. All of her sense of connections were distorted. When someone is sexually abused, there is an enormous breach of trust. NSPCC (2019) reported that over 90% of sexually abused children knew their abuser. The Office for National Statistics (2018) showed that 20% of women and 4% of men have experienced sexual assault since the age of 16: estimated 3.4 million female victims and 631,000 male victims in England and Wales. 5 in 6 victims (83%) did not report their experiences to the police. One of the reasons that victims don't report is because of a fear of not being believed, which is often a fear instilled by the perpetrators in the grooming process. Of course, the prevalence of sexual abuse is not only UK-based. Centres for Disease Control and Prevention (CDC) found that nearly 1 in 5 women in the USA is raped or sexually assaulted at some point in their lives. In some Asian, African and Middle East countries, that figure is even higher.

Francesca and I explored together the need that was being met by manipulating men into falling in lust with her; it was an attempt to be dominant, to have control and also to avoid vulnerability. Lust was powerful; love was dangerous (vulnerable). If she couldn't trust her father, who could she trust? I helped her re-frame her narrative, her unwanted sexual behaviours were not 'bad behaviours', they were attempts to recover and defend herself against future trauma. Gestalt Therapy informs us that

> in order to grow and develop people strive to maintain a balance between need gratification and tension elimination. Gestalt is a need-based approach, By stressing needs it places a very important focus on motivation (...) Working from their knowledge of the organism's tendency to self-regulation, Gestaltists assume that people know at some level what is good for them (2004, pp. 22–23).

Clarkson writes:

> One of the fundamental concepts of Gestalt theory is that the person is basically healthy and is striving for balance, health and growth (2004, p. 49).

This means that an unwanted behaviour may be an obstacle to self-actualisation but it is trying to heal a disturbance that is unresolved. Francesca understood it, but at the same time, she found it hard to accept the validation. I invited her to explore how she related to her anger. Was her anger a protection against vulnerability? Was it a way to protect her erotic world against further harm? In these conversations, I brought to her consciousness the different facets of connection. It made sense that she would create conflicts (connection with meaningful others) to keep her anger (connection with the world) to protect her erotic world (connection with self). What would her erotic world be if there wasn't any anger? It was a frightening thought for Francesca. I would like to stress that when we have these conversations with clients it is important that we don't prescribe implicit or explicit solutions such as *'you have to let go of anger'* or *'anger is bad'*. Many survivors of sexual abuse want to hold on to some anger, which is absolutely fine.

Francesca became more aware that she was meeting men based on her fantasy story but it was not a mutual fantasy with the men she chose. I said to her *'if you recruit a man to play a part in the story, it's easier if the man knows what part he is to play in which story'*.

However, in order to be honest with men about what she wanted out of her fantasy role plays required her to be vulnerable, a position that she found intolerable. Embarking on the conversations around vulnerability, she started to face the painful truth that she didn't love herself very much. She was once again putting some obstacles in between us and tried to create conflicts again so that she didn't have to engage in those conversations. She tried to be sarcastic; *'You want to talk about self-love because you're French, us British don't do that'*. Or she tried to criticise me *'Are you a hippy now?'* or *'You're only saying that because I'm paying you'*. I kept my unconditional positive regard, empathy and my patience. Eventually, in the consulting room, she began to have an actual experience of intimacy and vulnerability by allowing herself to be fully seen by me.

I could hear a negative cognition about herself in almost every sentence. She never quite realised how often she was putting herself down. She could recognise that she had learnt how to speak to herself that way because her parents taught her to adopt that negative language. Might there be another way of speaking to herself? She was kind and loving with her friends, could she do it for herself?

To prepare for trauma therapy, I first helped Francesca to anchor her safe place. She chose Bondi Beach in Sydney. It was a memory where she felt totally free and safe. We anchored it with all the positive somatic markers.

Having established an anchor, we moved to the trauma treatment. First, I asked her to bring a key trauma memory into headlines of only a few words.

1   Finishing dinner
2   Preparing for bed
3   Being in bed
4   Sexual abuse
5   He leaves the room
6   Waking up the next day
7   Going to school where I'm safer
8   Epilogue: I survived and now my father is nowhere near me.

When narrating the traumatic memory, the narrative should not be chronological, it should start with the epilogue to reinforce the psychological message: 'It's over now. I am safe now' (Rothschild, 2017). I asked Francesca to narrate using the word 'I' consistently.

After the epilogue, I asked Francesca to choose another section, not the worst part yet. She chose 'Preparing for bed'. In the narration of the traumatic memory, the key to safe trauma therapy is to keep clients one foot in the here-and-now as they remember the memory. I tell clients that I will interrupt them frequently. With each interruption, I ask here-and-now questions such as:

> *What are you feeling in your body now?*
> *Do you remember today's date although you are talking about a memory?*
> *Can you feel the chair you're sitting on?*

I also ask questions so that they can integrate different elements of the memory. The traumatic stress disappears when the narrative is well integrated. If a big emotion emerges, I stop and take the client back to their safe place straight away, and we talk about other things. Back and forth.

I interrupt for enquiries to solicit meaning-making.

> *What did you think then? What do you think now?*
> *Looking at the memory from your adult position, what do you make of this?*
> *What do you understand about this?*

Occasionally, I offer some psycho-education when appropriate, for example: *'it is normal to feel sexual pleasure even when the touch is unwanted'.* Or that *'it is normal that you loved your father even though he abused you. It was your father's responsibility to respect the boundaries, not yours'.*

Piece by piece, Francesca was able to feel more compassionate to her Inner Child and process the anger towards her father for his abuse, her mother for being inadequate, other adults around her who didn't protect her, possibly even turned a blind eye. She was able to start having a new meaning to these stories.

I used a 'Back to Sender' guided visualisation to consolidate the process of her trauma therapy. I suggested Francesca imagined that all the heavy things she was carrying were actually her father's, she could put them all in a parcel and send them back. Penny Parks (1990, 1994) offers a wide range of visualisation techniques to help recover from childhood sexual abuse.

Throughout the process, I enquired how she was doing in between each session. I noticed that she reported upping her self-care by herself. For example, she paid more attention to how she ate, and she allowed herself to sleep more. Slowly, I could see that she was filling her pie of life without me addressing it explicitly. This is when I can see how our instinct for survival is always intact, we can naturally do things that are good for us when we have enough of a nurturing frame.

Bessel Van Der Kolk explains that healing from trauma is owning your self, which involves:

> (1) finding a way to become calm and focused, (2) learning to maintain that calm in response to images, thoughts, sounds, or physical sensations that remind you of the past, (3) finding a way to be fully alive in the present and engaged with people around you, (4) not having to keep secrets from yourself, including secrets about the ways that you have managed to survive (2014, pp. 203–204).

In the context of CSB, the fourth part is essential as often the survival strategies were sexual compulsivity.

As Francesca progressed in therapy, not without its bumps on the road, she was then able to make contact with her deep grief for her lost childhood. She never had good models for being a woman in the world, for relationships, for love, for intimacy. Grieving is a meaning making process, just as much as trauma therapy. Francesca was transforming before my eyes, slowly, changing her script of '*I'm OK – You're not OK*' to '*I'm OK – You might be OK*'.

She was now ready to connect meaningfully with her body and her erotic. I proposed an exercise of self-sensate focus, where she could enjoy the pleasure of her own touch without any judgements. It was challenging for Francesca at first because she never allowed herself to feel erotic without the attraction of another. I stressed to Francesca that feeling someone else wanted and desired her sexually was a great feeling, and there was nothing wrong with that. But connecting with our own body and our own pleasure was a totally different erotic experience.

Later, she discovered that she had a great erotic time when the men actually agreed to take part in her role plays; she met all the six principles of sexual health. Francesca reported no more compulsion to her sexual behaviours. We discussed Dr Gurney's '*conditions for good sex*' triangle: psychological arousal, physical touch and being in the moment, which helped Francesca stay in touch with her eroticism. Gurney writes that the personality trait that predicts sexual satisfaction is conscientiousness. The role play Francesca enjoyed were carefully planned and therefore conscientious. She now realised that what she previously thought of as '*weird*' was actually the very thing that enhanced her sex life.

Anna

I can summarise quite simply the therapy with Anna: normalising her sexual behaviours, her non-heteronormative vision of her life and empowering her to continue living a life that aligns with her authentic self. I used a person-centred approach combined with psychosexual and relationship dialogues to help Anna with reducing her society-induced shame and feeling more congruent with her authentic self. We also worked with her body posture, as standing tall also helped with countering her shame. As a result, she became more confident, without needing to apologise to anybody for who she was. Before therapy, she knew intellectually that it was ok to be a woman and not wanting children or a monogamous partner, but after therapy, she knew it in her gut too. She was more mindful about her Connection Circles and gained clarity about who 'her tribe' was. When she was more connected to her own people and less concerned about the people that did not share her values, her shame disappeared, and she no longer had preoccupying thoughts about her sexual behaviours. She stopped thinking that her behaviours were out of control. Anna's therapy is an example of how swift a CSB treatment can be. Anna didn't actually have a sexual behaviour problem but her distress was informed by her shame born out of heteronormativity. Once she re-aligned herself with who she was, the distress she felt about her sexual behaviours disappeared.

Gay men

Peter

Exploring Peter's pie of life brought forth his lack of a sense of belonging. I encouraged him to start with something small and achievable. He joined a gay running club; it doubled up as a social event to meet new non-sexual friends. He struggled with sexual urges towards some of his running buddies. I introduced to him the four elements (Air, Earth, Water, Fire) for his urge reduction and impulse control, which he used successfully.

Betty Martin's website on the 'Wheel of Consent' brought much clarity to Peter regarding mutual pleasure and how to give and receive touch. He became aware that gifting his body for other's pleasures was a potent turn-on for him, which he added in his Erotic Template; touching others for his pleasure was erotically less intense.

I decided to introduce the Inner Child visualisation so that Peter could hug and nurture his Inner Child. It was reparative of his traumatic experience of his father scolding him for his sexuality. I used some ACT methods (Hayes et al., 2012) to address accepting his sexuality and healing the negative impact of his father's homophobia. Peter learnt how to make a commitment with himself for self-compassion and self-care, which was previously unknown to him. It was a challenging time because he felt shame for talking about his father in a negative light. I stressed to him that this work was not about blaming his father but healing the wounds of some of his father's behaviours that currently impacted on his life. I also invited

Peter to think about the impact of homophobia not only coming from his father but from society too. Growing up in a heteronormative world can create a sense of self, that is *'hopelessly flawed'*, as noticed by Joe Kort (2018). Kort says that even if LGBTQ people did not experience direct homophobic violence, they experience vicarious trauma from various media reporting hate crimes. Indeed, if we are attuned to it, we hear LGBTQ people being hunted and killed around the world regularly.

In line with the honesty element of the six principles of sexual health, I encouraged some honest conversations over Peter's choice of monogamy as he seemed to have agreed to it with Carlos but without thinking about it properly. He thought monogamy was the 'Gold Standard', a myth that could precipitate erotic conflicts, as well documented by Perel (2017). He was reluctant to bring this subject to his partner because he didn't want Carlos to ask uncomfortable questions but he was willing to have conversations about doing something different sexually. They discussed taking turns in bringing some dominance and submissive play in their sex life; Peter was surprised that Carlos, whom he previously thought of as 'Vanilla', was quite happy to explore this light kink. It made Peter aware that he had had an image of Carlos that was largely based on assumptions. Now that they were having more explicit conversations, they were both able to meet Peter's sensation seeking, and therefore resolved some of the erotic conflict. Peter's perception of his relationship had been split; Carlos was 'the good gay' (vanilla) and he was the 'dirty gay' (promiscuous). Hearing Carlos being open to light kink helped build a bridge between the two. I recommended the book *'Re-writing the Rules'* by Meg-John Barker (2018). Their book is labelled as *'anti self-help'* as it encourages introspection instead of tips, which both Peter and Carlos found helpful.

Peter's split thinking resided within himself too. Some internalised homo-negativity was set in a deprivation script (*I must follow the straight and narrow path of being a good boyfriend*) which paradoxically set up what Peter described as *'gluttony'* (*I want to binge on sex*). The underlying conflicts was that he felt *'obliged'* to be monogamous because *'that's what good gay men do'* but also to be promiscuous because *'that's what all gay men do'*. Peter's sexuality lived in a confusing world of contradictions between the *'good gay man'* and *'the desirable gay man'*. Giving one up would mean a tremendous loss. I asked if there was a possibility to have a vision of a gay man being desirable and a good boyfriend. With this question, we returned to his erotic transference; he responded that I was that vision. He assumed that I was *'sexually open-minded'*, given the job I do, and he perceived me as the *'perfect balance of warmth and sexuality'*. I asked him what his fantasy about me was. He said that he thought I was married, in an open relationship, a little kinky, living in a trendy apartment in Central London. It was quite a detailed image. I asked him if it was an image that he wanted for himself or what he wanted in his partner. He said he wanted that for himself.

The conversation thus shifted from an erotic transference to one of re-parenting. His father had not been able to guide him with his sexual and relational maturity, but he now looked to me to be his guide as I represented the less confusing, and perhaps more realistic, picture of what a gay man can be; not the romantic gay wedding ads, nor the sex clubbing, but the in-between; an authentic person holding both the relational and sexual space.

I suggested that he looked into how he could meet his LGBTQ commu-nity from one person to another rather than a sexual object to another to replicate the benefit of what he was getting out of our therapeutic re-lationship. He eventually decided to go to London Pride for the first time in his life. In the next session he told me that it was '*an amazing experience*'; he noticed the large diversity of gay men to be young, old, thin, big, disabled, friendly, sexual, non-sexual, and so on. He felt he had a place in the com-munity, he felt part of a '*new family*', for the first time. This experiment seemed to be one of the major turning points of his therapy because he found his sense of belonging.

By owning his story and being in full awareness of his childhood messages and rectifying them, he was able to make more adult-based decisions for himself. In one session, Peter said: '*I had a lot of fun in sex clubs, and I will continue to enjoy these memories, but I can let it go now, I don't need it in my life anymore*'. He believed he would suit polyamory better, as per his relational desire discussed at the beginning of therapy, but he didn't want to let go of Carlos whom he assumed was only interested in monogamy. In his process of maturity, he was aware that he needed the balance of making the compromises that were acceptable to him and knowing the values of his Erotic Template that could not be compromised. I cautioned him not to make a promise to Carlos if he didn't think he could keep it. He felt more courageous to have a con-versation with his partner and, once again, he realised that his assumption was wrong. Carlos did value monogamy but he wasn't so rigid about it. I proposed to Peter to think about '*monogam-ish*', a term coined by Dan Savage, author of '*The Commitment*' (2005). It helped them both agree on acceptable compro-mises; Peter reported to me that discussing their '*monogam-ish*' boundaries actually deepened their connection. I informed Peter that he and Carlos had the right to change their mind about their arrangement, and they could have an-nual reviews. Peter had a much better grounding of his sense of autonomy and he felt he now made his voice heard in his relationship.

Peter reported no more compulsivity in his sexual behaviours as they were now congruent with the six principles of sexual health. Although Carlos noticed Peter was the original instigator of change due to his requests of honest conversations, he never knew about his sexual behaviours with other men. Perel (2017) challenges the notion of transparency:

> On more than one occasion, I've seen honesty do more harm than good, leaving me to ask, can lying sometimes be protective? (...) Sometimes

silence is caring. Before you unload your guilt onto an unsuspecting partner, consider, whose well-being are you really thinking of? Is your soul-cleansing as selfless as it appears? And what is your partner supposed to do with this information? (2017, pp. 130–1).

Peter accepted that he would have to live with his secret, but he also felt proud of himself for learning to be in a conscious relationship with Carlos, which made them both happier. In the process, he healed much of his homophobic childhood.

Chemsex

George

Most clients struggling with Chemsex don't want to be labelled 'addicts', for good reasons. These words are loaded with stigma. Most clients describe their struggle with Chemsex as compulsive. Using the right terminology is very important for all populations to avoid shame, but they are more particularly important when working with the LGBTQ community because words have forever been used to pathologise them.

It is tempting for the psychotherapist to be concerned about overdose and to want to rush the client into abstinence. Sexual behaviours during Chemsex are loaded with shame because participants have unprotected sex with strangers, they have sex with people they don't find attractive, they have sex with multiple partners at once and they sometimes don't remember how they had sex, which becomes a consent issue. The multi-layered shame makes clients sensitive to the psychotherapist's judgements. As soon as the client feels a hint of judgement from the therapist, they will disengage. At the beginning, rather than discussing abstinence from drugs, it is important to have a conversation about 'safer Chemsex'. If psychotherapists invite clients with these enquiries first, the client will feel that the therapist is on their side, rather than a Critical Parent Ego State.

The study by Sewell et al. (2019) indicates that behavioural change in Chemsex is observed when there is the right approach, suggesting that an exploration of the behaviours and consequences in a non-judgmental dialogue encourages a reduction in Chemsex behaviours. But it is not all. Studies by Stardust et al. (2018) and Burgess et al. (2018) both highlight the importance of community, peer-led support group for harm-reduction. This makes sense, given that internalised homo-negativity and minority stress lurk underneath Chemsex. Meeting other gay and bisexual men and MSM, and having meaningful conversations together, away from all the noise of the gay scene and social media, a haven of honesty, truth and humanity, can be powerfully reparative. With this in mind, I signposted George to the Soho clinic 56 Dean

Street, which is the NHS' best clinic in Chemsex support, as well as the resources available on David Stuart's website.

George reported that he never had the chance to talk about his erotic mind in such detail before therapy. Doing so with me, someone with whom sexual contact is impossible was an important experience for him because the boundaries were clear and therefore he felt safe. As soon as he felt supported by me, he asked me to help him with stopping taking drugs. I didn't jump on his request, which would send the implicit psychological message 'I've been waiting for this'. Instead, I asked him why he wanted to stop. I encouraged him to tell me about all the things he enjoyed about Chemsex and what he would miss if he did stop. George felt strong somatic activations with his Chemsex memories, which he called '*anticipatory horniness*'. He described the Chemsex parties as the only place where he could totally let himself go and feel completely accepted by others. I told him that it sounded like a lot to give up. I asked him if he was really sure he wanted to give it up. George thought about it for a moment. He said '*no*', then he felt relief for being honest with himself: '*I think I should give up because it's not good for me. But, you're right. It's not giving up the drugs, it's giving up all the good stuff that comes with it. Maybe that's why I never managed to stop before*'. Admitting his ambivalence about this was a great and honest place to start. We could still discuss behavioural change with what Stuart and Weymann call '*Chemsex Care Planning*' (2015) as discussed in Part 2. Clients can experiment what it is like not to do Chemsex for a short period of time without asking themselves to permanently give up all the good things associated with it.

George had difficulty engaging with Mindfulness. I reassured him that there wasn't right or wrong ways of doing therapy, it was just about finding the strategies that worked for him. Promoting clients' autonomy in not doing a proposed method by the therapist is just as valuable as teaching them those skills. George realised that his emotional regulation strategies had to be dynamic. He got on better with muscle tensing and jogging. Over time, he started to develop new interests he didn't know he had, such as redecorating his flat and DIY, which provided him with a good, pleasurable meaningful interest on weekends, taking himself away from the urges of Chemsex, which reduced his sexual compulsivity.

Although, on the surface, it appeared that George was at his most vulnerable on Thursdays because it was when he had the stronger urges about doing Chemsex, feeling bad about himself on his come down stage from Mondays to Wednesdays were his most emotionally vulnerable times as it was when he was feeding his low self-esteem. The stronger the self-loathing, the stronger was the need for Chemsex. With the drugs, George was going from self-loathing to full acceptance instantly. When he realised that Thursdays weren't really the problem, he thought for himself that perhaps he should reduce his come-down period. I asked him how he might achieve that. '*Perhaps taking less drugs*'. George was able to create his own care plan framed with 'experimenting' which took away the notion of failure or success. Doing so in this manner promoted self-reliance, trusting that clients have their own wisdom when provided with the right space to access it. It also promoted developing George's own sexual health-oriented thinking.

George's plan was unsuccessful on that weekend. He came to therapy with more self-loathing: '*I didn't do as I planned. I relapsed. I'm broken. I'm hopeless*'. I slowed him down and reminded him of the frame: the care plan was an experiment. Experiments don't always go as planned. Instead of thinking of a relapse, I encouraged George to think of it as a '*Learning Event*'. When George started to think about it carefully, instead of labelling the whole weekend as '*failure*' he said '*Actually I remembered some of our discussions on safer Chemsex and I did take more care with it. I didn't inject. And I was more aware of what I enjoyed about it.*' When George thought that indeed, there was a slight change to his behaviours, he became more hopeful. Together we brainstormed different ideas. He settled with planning something for Saturday afternoon that he would look forward to. It couldn't be anything high energy though. He thought about having his favourite comforting drink, a hot chocolate, and his favourite Netflix programme. How about Saturday afternoon being the wonderful quality time of hot chocolate and Netflix, after the high horniness of Friday night? He was up for that!

The following week, George was beaming because he was successful in maintaining his plan. As he was navigating his own Chemsex care plan and he gradually increased his drug-free period. We continued to discuss what he would miss if he stopped the drugs completely. He started to feel the fear of being lonely and the inability to have sober sex. He associated sober sex with 'boring' sex now. I normalised his experience with the analogy of food '*it's like eating spicy food all the time, then food without it can taste bland*'.

Managing urges is crucial but it is not the only resource needed. George and I discussed his friendship circle. He realised that he only knew people involved in the Chemsex scene. Moving away from it meant a great loss of friendship and identity as demonstrated in the study by Smith and Tasker (2018) which found Chemsex was associated with positive gay identity gain. Loneliness was connected to '*feeling different*' in childhood as well as homophobia. The fear of loneliness was a fear of never being loved apart from when he was high, and the fear of losing his current sex life was distressing to him. George became aware that he was living with multiple fears. George's vision of the future revealed both an excitement to be away from the Chemsex scene and a fear of not knowing what life could be like without it.

When George successfully spent an entire weekend without Chemsex, he felt scared rather than proud. '*I slept a lot that weekend, but I was so bored. I felt so lonely. I realised that my life is empty without Chemsex*'. We talked about his pie of life. He wanted to focus on friendship and sex. Kunelaki

(2019) defines sober sex as *'present sex where no drugs (chemsex) or fantasies are involved, and the connection between body and mind is maintained'*. Kunelaki offers clinical guidelines to help clients towards sober sex, focusing on mindful masturbation to start with. George felt that it was a good introduction to a new sex life, it was less frightening than experimenting with others at this stage.

I proposed to George to do the Traffic Light Exercise on what he wanted for himself for his sex and relationship life after Chemsex. He described wanting to be in a sexual and romantic relationship with one person. He wanted a diverse sex life with this one person, including room to experiment with some kink. He wanted a sex life completely free from Chemsex. And he wanted more gay friends. He was happy to have role plays in the amber section, depending on his partner. George's care plan was reviewed regularly, now including his Traffic Lights. We discussed the six principles of sexual health. He realised how difficult it was to meet all sexual health principles in Chemsex, so the party events became hard work rather than fun.

When we revisited George's childhood, he got in touch with the pain of feeling rejected by his parents, a pain he hadn't felt in a long time. George found it hard to validate it because his parents weren't overtly abusive. I said to George: *'pain is pain. There isn't a type of pain that is more legitimate than another'*. We spent many sessions discussing in details the dismissed pain of experiencing his father preferring his brother because they were both into football, the impact of his critical mother, the needing to hide who he really was throughout school, the guilt for taking advantage of a shy girl to pretend to be her straight boyfriend, disregarding her feelings. With compassion-focused dialogues, we brought to the surface all the emotions that were repressed: the shame, the fears, the anger, the sadness, the confusions and so on. With each step of the way, I challenged George when I heard some negative cognition about himself. I helped him re-frame his mistakes as *'strategies for survival'*. He was able to see his story again from a different perspective, he was able to observe his own Inner Child being really lost in a heteronormative world, with little guidance. Slowly, my walking by his side naturally faded, replaced by his Adult Self walking by the side of his Inner Child. It was a moving process to witness. By then, his Chemsex behaviours fully stopped and he no longer experienced sexual compulsivity. But the work wasn't completely done. His pie of life was still in deficit. He found it difficult to engage with other people in the LGBTQ scene and he still often felt lonely. This was concerning to me because it meant he could still be vulnerable to return to the Chemsex scene. Having a strong sense of connection and belonging was paramount to leaving Chemsex truly behind.

I did not foresee Phase 3 being the most difficult phase for George. But indeed it was. My colleague Juliette Clancy wrote a blog *The Shame of Loneliness*, a useful piece of reflection for us all. Clancy opens the conversation on thinking of loneliness as a guest in our lives as part of our human existence rather than something shameful that should be banished. It was helpful for George thinking about loneliness differently. He was a man enjoying DIY, hot chocolate, Netflix and in-depth meaningful conversations. This image did not fit the *'sexy gay'* which *'should be'* hot, young, hypersexual, have a perfect body, successful in every way, partying and always wanted. Outside of my consulting room, he could not find the courage to connect with others in the gay scene. The gay social apps were bold, mostly focused on sex and partying. I realised that the biggest block was not George's psychological state but the harsh gay hook-up scene. The LGBTQ community is one which survived much trauma, but in its survival strategy, it can be unforgiving of vulnerability and imperfections. George didn't want to return to the Chemsex scene. He didn't connect with the gay scene. What was left for him? I proposed to George that perhaps he could meet gay men in other places. George agreed with me but didn't do anything about it for months. The anxiety of rejection was high. But one day, George took the plunge, he registered for a gay tennis club. I never experienced him so anxious. His first meetings with the gay tennis club went well. George was so relieved he cried in session. Going through this major hurdle was the last piece of the pie for George. From that point on, the rest of his life fell into place effortlessly. He continued with gay tennis every week, making new good friends. He then connected with a gay hiking group and made more meaningful friendships. After his recovery from Chemsex, I saw George flourishing before my eyes. Making meaningful connections, increasing his sense of belonging and well-being. Later, he challenged himself to connect with a hobby group that was not gay-specific. He realised he was accepted by the heterosexual population too, and made friends with them too, which healed his internalised homo-negativity further. Eventually, he met a man whom he started dating. George was reluctant to stop therapy as he wanted some relationship advice from me through his dating stage. I could have given him many dating tips but I didn't feel it was the right thing for him. I simply said: *'You know yourself very well now. Be yourself as fully as you can be, and you will know what to do'*. George felt a bit short-changed in that session but he understood my message; living a life in autonomy required trusting himself. I was right, he didn't need any tips from me; his date became his boyfriend. I did help George with building up confidence to pace his boyfriend in taking it slowly sexually, taking the time to enjoy every minute of sober sex. At that point, George decided to finish therapy. It was the right time, indeed.

Queer population: kink community

Pascale

I noticed that it was difficult for Pascale to be present in the consulting room. They would often dissociate by glazing over, stopping speaking for a long time. I spent much time with them to bring them back in the here-and-now and introducing emotional regulation. In their moments of dissociation, I asked them to clap their hands, stand up and name what they saw in my consulting room. I wanted to work towards Pascale being more aware of their body. I introduced an exercise of mindful self-touching. It didn't work much, it was hard for them to feel anything on their body. They didn't think therapy was going to work and they started to display behaviours shrugging their shoulders thinking '*why am I even here?*'. We were both walking in the dark. I took the opportunity of this difficult start of therapy to spend more time with emotional regulation, including dual awareness, which was particularly useful for Pascale even though they were still thinking therapy wasn't going to work. Gently, I tried to explore what happened in 2012 because it was when the symptoms started. I asked them to describe one event in 2012 when they felt distressed or numb. Pascale's mind came up with a peculiar memory. They were stepping out of the tube onto the platform and stumbled across a person dressed in a furry suit, it was to do with the London Olympics promotion. Pascale remembered feeling startled, their heart rate going up, their stomach dropping and then instant dissociation.

Pascale started to remember, it was a really blurry faint memory, but the feeling in their body was strong: they were sexually abused whilst holding a teddy bear. The person dressed in a furry suit was the somatic marker that alerted Pascale's amygdala that it was dangerous as it was linked to a significant trauma. They remembered that the teddy bear smelt of peanuts, which Pascale thought was a strange thing to remember, but interestingly, they said they were allergic to peanuts. I brought them back to the here-and-now again as I didn't want them to go into a full-blown flashback. Using dual awareness, I made sure Pascale understood that whilst they were remembering some things, they were also here, in my consulting room, in safety. I paced Pascale and slowed them down because when clients start to remember some memories, it might be the tip of the iceberg in a series of deeply traumatic events. I told Pascale that we will not make assumptions about what did or didn't happen in their past, but we will process whatever their body is holding. I reassured Pascale that they didn't need to remember everything in order to heal. I validated to them that not remembering was a good strategy.

We spent a few sessions on emotional regulation again, not addressing the trauma, as we needed to pace it. In one session Pascale took another deep breath. '*I was seven years old, I went to see a psychologist.*' Pascale's parents were always concerned about their children being perfect, and each time there was a 'problem', they sent their children to a psychologist. I noticed Pascale started getting agitated, breathing quicker. I put on the brakes at that moment, grounding them back to the here-and-now. They wanted to talk about it, but I paced them to avoid re-traumatisation. We spent time in Pascale's internal safe place until their nervous system was calmer.

The week after, Pascale reported having many vivid disturbing dreams with the teddy bear. They used the emotional regulation we practiced in sessions on waking from these dreams, which were helpful. As the smell was one of the memories that came back up, we discussed that they could use an essential oil smell to counter-act that, as an extra emotional regulation strategy. They opted for rosemary.

The dreams were of the teddy bear suffocating them. They would wake up in the middle of the night in sweats gasping for air. They noticed that at that moment, they also felt sexual as well as distressed. They told me that they couldn't help but masturbate fast and slapping their vulva in order to orgasm before going back to sleep. I asked them if it was soothing or distressing to do so. They said that it calmed them down, I did not challenge this but we discussed how to add extra strategies when waking up at night. One of them was going to the bathroom and pouring cold water on their wrists, which also calmed them.

In the following session, Pascale said: *'Nounours'* (it's the French word for teddy bear). *'The psychologist wasn't very inventive, he called his teddy bear Nounours.'* The more Pascale remembered, the more we processed their memories, in a range of interventions, including somatic trauma therapy, EMDR and EFT. Gradually, Pascale was able to feel their body again.

The following Summer, they visited their parents and asked about the psychologist. Their mother cried. Two years after they stopped seeing the psychologist, there was a complaint made against him, and he was found guilty. Their mother's guilt at sending her own children to a sex offender was so big that she stayed silent and never talked about it. Pascale's mother explained the psychologist committed suicide before he went to prison. Their mother prayed their children were spared from the psychologist's abuse, but, confronted with Pascale's questions, their mother had to face the worst. Was sending them to the psychologist the cause of one of her children ending their life? Pascale's mother apologised profoundly. Pascale felt empathy, they could see she was truly sorry.

Slowly, bit by bit, Pascale was able to process whatever they remembered about the trauma, piecing together all the elements that had not been processed before; the context, the story, sensory memories, and meaning. As they healed their trauma, Pascale started to understand that their trauma reaction in 2012 caused their dissociation that pushed them outside of their BDSM boundaries. They took time to enjoy mindful masturbation as they could feel their body again. They were ready once again to engage in their loved BDSM scene. Pascale's BDSM activities didn't change from before the eruption of their trauma symptoms. They were happy and clear that their BDSM turn-on was not associated with trauma. Pascale had no more trauma symptoms, they reported no more sexual compulsion, and they enjoyed a vibrant sex life that matched their Erotic Template and met the six principles of sexual health.

People of religious beliefs

Terry

Terry felt ashamed for talking about his parents in a negative light. He was defensive with me each time I asked a question about his childhood: '*it's not my parents' fault, it's me who has a dark side*'. His loop of shame was strong. I enquired about the pleasure of his weekly non-sexual massages. He answered with tears, which turned into a sob. Eventually, when he caught his breath, Terry muttered: '*I was never touched as a child*'. Terry never got to be soothed, never hugged, and he was told it was for his own good.

As an adult, it became a routine to go to a masseuse to soothe himself from busy, stressful weeks. Claire was not tactile either, she was always busy with appearance, cleaning the house, appearing good, but emotionally cold. If he tried to touch her, she would tell him he pestered her, and he should keep his hands to himself. His wife allowed him to have sex with her to have children, and after childbirth sex disappeared; she always had better things to do.

Sexual betrayal is often understood as having sex outside of the committed relationship, but it is not always validated as the non-consensual withdrawal of sex from a relationship. Did his wife commit sexual betrayal too? Re-framing this, I helped Terry think that he wasn't the only person bringing a problem in his marriage. He described Claire's behaviours as constantly putting him down. She also threatened to destroy his reputation at Church. These were abusive behaviours although Terry did not evaluate them as such.

I asked Terry if it was appropriate for me to deliver some psycho-education on pornography, as I didn't want to be disrespectful of his religious values. He agreed. He understood the research on pornography, it made him feel better about himself. He didn't think of himself as a '*sinner*' any longer. But he did not want to divorce Claire. She did not want divorce either as it was against their Christian values. I suggested to him to do the Traffic Lights exercise and explain to her that touch is a core part of his being and that deprivation of it was not ok for him. After the discovery of pornography watching, Claire made sure that Terry understood she would not have sex with him again. He stayed assertive and invited her to a brainstorm on how he wanted to be sexual. They both agreed that avoiding divorce meant that they had to make compromises. They both consented to a different 'contract'. He became honest about his non-sexual massages and Claire agreed to them. After our normalising conversations on pornography and the fact that Claire put sex off the table, he asked if he could watch pornography as long as it was done in the room upstairs at certain times. There would be no more expectations of the two of them being sexual. She refused. With my guidance, he asked her what would be the best way he could meet his sexual needs that she could consent to. Claire was once again assertive with Terry that she was not interested in sex and she did not understand why Terry was still interested in sex. She continued to be angry with him for having watched pornography and she told him that she would be angry forever about it, Terry told me in tears.

The six principles of sexual health require honesty and shared values. Continuing to do a sexual activity against Claire's consent would be a breach of these and he would continue to feel bad about himself. On the other hand, Claire left him no room to meet his sexual needs, which are his human and sexual right.

Our sessions had been reparative for him, being in a truly safe place where he could be seen and heard fully with no judgements or expectations. My therapy with Terry was mostly person-centred (Rogers, 1961), which was the healing agent for him. However, our therapeutic reach had limitations. We could not ask Claire to change her important values. Terry knew that he could only change himself in the attempt to change the system of his marriage. Unfortunately, Claire responded with more anger, which made the space less safe for Terry. After many sessions of my holding, one day, Terry came to his own conclusion that perhaps he needed to end his marriage even though it was against his Christian values. I asked him to think about it carefully before making any move towards it. Was it what he really wanted? Had he thought about all the possible consequences? Terry said that as a result of our sessions, he became acutely aware that it was not ok to be denied any way to meet his sexuality and that there was some domestic abuse going on. He said that he tried all he could to resolve issues with Claire but she never budged. After quite a few more sessions of thinking and reflecting, he made the decision to move out. He was terrified at Claire's reactions. To his surprise, she did not become rageful. She told him that she was pleased he took the decision instead of her because she did not have to live with the fact that it was she who broke the sanctity of marriage. In reflection, Terry thought that she probably stopped loving him a long time ago and engineered a separation that would induce him breaking up so that she could stay *'clean'* with her faith. In the year that followed, I helped Terry process his tremendous grief and disappointment at losing his marriage and I supported him through every step of his separation and divorce.

The reconstruction for Terry was to do the psychological version of the Japanese art *'Kinsukuroi'*, the golden repair. I continued with the Rogerian trajectory of therapy and added some ACT-based self-compassion and commitment of self-care (Harris, 2019), to help him find peace with being a Christian divorcee as well as embracing his erotic world. I validated that it was ok to still love Claire and to cherish all their good memories together, and it was also ok to stay true to himself with her not fitting with his life any longer. His faith for his religion had remained intact whilst having a new view of his sexuality. As soon as Terry moved out and was away from

Claire's disapproval, he no longer felt compulsive with his pornography watching and sexual behaviours.

He met another woman from his religious community, a divorcee too. He made sure he established the principles of sexual health with her from the beginning to start a new relationship on the right footing. Pornography was acceptable in his new relationship but on the basis of *'don't ask, don't tell'*. Terry found it good enough for him, especially because he also got plenty of touch and satisfying sex with her.

References

Barker, M.J. (2018). *Rewriting the rules: an anti self-help guide to love, sex and relationships*, 2nd ed. Abingdon, Oxon: Routledge.

Berne, E. (2009). *Transactional analysis in psychotherapy*. California: Snowball Publishing.

Burgess et al. (2018). Re-wired: treatment and peer support for men who have sex with men who use methamphetamine. *Sexual Health*, 15, 157–159.

Centres for Disease Control and Prevention (CDC). The National Intimate and Sexual Violence Survey (NISVS). [Available Online]: https://www.cdc.gov/violenceprevention/datasources/nisvs/index.html.

Clancy, J. Website. *Thoughts from the couch: the shame of loneliness*. [Available Online]: http://www.julietteclancycounselling.com/thoughts-from-the-couch-the-shame-of-loneliness/.

Clarkson, P. (2004). *Gestalt counselling in action*, 3rd ed. London: Sage.

Fairburn, C.G. (2013). *Overcoming binge eating*, 2nd ed. New York: Guilford Press.

Greenberger, D. and Padesky, C.A. (1995). *Mind over mood*. New York: The Guildford Press.

Gurney, K. (2020). *Mind the gap: the truth about desire and how to futureproof your sex life*. London: Headline Publishing Group.

Harris, R. (2019). *ACT made simple*, 2nd ed. Oakland, CA: New Harbinger.

Hayes, S.C., Strosahl, K.D. and Wilson, K.G. (2012). *Acceptance and commitment therapy: the process and practice of mindful change*, 2nd ed. New York: The Guildford Press.

Kellogg, S. (2015). *Transformational chairwork*. Lanham, Maryland: Rowman & Littlefield.

Kort, J. (2018). *LGBTQ clients in therapy: clinical issues and treatment strategies*. New York: W.W. Norton & Company.

Kunelaki, R. (2019). What is sober sex and how to achieve it. *Drugs and Alcohol Today*. https://doi.org/10.1108/DAT-11–2018-0064.

Martin, B. The Wheel of Consent website. [Available Online]: https://bettymartin.org/videos/.

Morin, J. (1995). *The erotic mind*. New York: HarperCollins.

NSPCC. (2019). Statistics briefing: child sexual abuse. [Available Online]: https://learning.nspcc.org.uk/media/1710/statistics-briefing-child-sexual-abuse.pdf.

Office for National Statistics. (2018). Sexual offences in England and Wales: year ending March 2017. [Available Online]: https://www.ons.gov.uk/peoplepopulationandcommunity/crimeandjustice/articles/sexualoffencesinenglandandwales/yearendingmarch2017.

Parks, P. (1990). *Rescuing the 'inner child': therapy for adults sexually abused as children*. London: Condor Book Souvenir Press (E&A) Ltd.

Parks, P. (1994). *Parks inner child therapy*. London: Condor Book Souvenir Press (E&A) Ltd.

Perel, E. (2017). *The state of affairs: rethinking infidelity*. London: Yellow Kite.

Rogers, C.R. (1961). *On becoming a person: a therapist's view of psychotherapy*. London: Constable & Robinson.

Rothschild, B. (2017). *The body remembers, volume 2. Revolutionizing trauma treatment*. New York: W.W.Norton & Company.

Savage, D. (2005). *The commitment*. London: Plume, Penguin Group.

Sewell, et al. (2019). Changes in Chemsex and sexual behaviour over time, among a cohort of MSM in London and Brighton: findings from the AURAH2 Study. *International Journal of Drug Policy,* 68, 54–61.

Shepherd, T. (2018). *Cognitive behavioural therapy*. Wroclaw, Poland: CreateSpace Independent Publishing Platform.

Smith, V. and Tasker, F. (2018). Gay men's chemsex survival stories. *Sexual Health Journal*, 15, 116–122.

Stardust et al. (2018). A community-led, harm-reduction approach to chemsex: case study from Australia's largest gay city. *Sexual Health*, 15, 179–181.

Stuart, D. Website [Available online]: https://www.davidstuart.org.

Stuart, D. and Weymann, J. (2015). ChemSex and care planning: one year in practice. *HIV Nursing,* 15, 24–28.

Tonkin, L. *Growing around grief*. [Available online]: http://www.loistonkin.com/growing-around-grief.html.

Van Der Kolk, B. (2014). *The body keeps the score: mind, brain and body in the transformation of trauma*. London: Allen Lane, Penguin Group.

Chapter 14

Working online

Since the COVID-19 pandemic working online has been a big feature of our psychotherapy profession and it is likely to remain a more popular method of therapy. In my own experience, I find that we can do deep relational and connection-focused therapeutic work online as efficiently as in-person therapy. Working online with clients who have compulsive sexual behaviours offer both challenges and opportunities.

Safe and confidential space

When working online, the responsibility of confidentiality is shared between the client and the therapist as the client has to make sure they are not overheard as much as we have to make sure that our space is private. For some, it can be a challenge because they might live in a flat with thin walls and hearing their partner and children in the next room will make clients feel uncomfortable. Some opt to have sessions in their car as it can be the best confidential space. Most people somehow find a way to have a safe place for themselves.

Appropriate space and clothing

The behavioural etiquette for online therapy should be the same as face-to-face therapy whereby it is not appropriate for a client to have therapy if they are not properly dressed. We need to discuss that it is not a good idea to have therapy if they are lying down on their bed, or drinking alcohol. It may be obvious to us but it may not be for some clients. People might think that being home means that they can be more relaxed. An exploration of their transference examining what was behind the therapy etiquette-breaching behaviours will be fertile grounds for their therapeutic process.

The online disinhibition effect

Suler (2004) teaches us that clients may be likely to disclose more materials and quicker than in traditional face-to-face therapy when having online therapy. It can be benign when clients feel they can open up more and share more things, including some secret fantasies and sexual feelings or behaviours they felt bad about. The disinhibition effect can be good in the context of CSB because it can actually speed up the work. However, be aware that the disinhibition effect works both ways. Therapist, too, can ask more direct questions and poke at people's private world too soon.

The online disinhibition effect may also be toxic. This is when people feel ok to insult or threaten someone, the kind of behaviours they would never do face-to-face. It is rare that this happens in the context of therapy, but we should keep this in mind.

The online space of therapy and sexual activity

Offering therapy for CSB online brings an interesting dynamic between the therapist and the client, especially if much of the client's unwanted sexual behaviours are online-based. For some clients, using the same device to see their therapist and their sex workers might just be too confusing. They might want to have two separate devices. But for some other people, it may be valuable to explore the transference that emerge out of meeting online. During the several COVID-19 lockdowns, much of our lives were online: work, social, therapy and sex. Somehow, we had to compartmentalise the different areas of our lives whilst being on one device, in one physical place. For some clients, having therapy on the same device as their sex lives might be an opportunity to desensitise the sexual behaviours and make it more *'normal'*: a space where the behaviours can be talked through, a place of various soothing, grounding and calm, a place where clients can make more sense of their sexual behaviours.

What we don't see

When providing online therapy, we have to be more aware of what we don't see. Might there be someone else in the room? This would be rare in the context of CSB therapy. But sometimes, we may encounter clients whose partner is controlling and abusive and they might want to control what is said or not said to their therapist.

Therapists need to make more enquiries about what is going on with the client's body. Do they feel their feet on the floor? Do they contort their body because of anxiety? Making those enquiries will help clients be more aware of their body language and offer an investigation of what is going on for them.

What we see

Therapists will see their clients' own space, and they will see ours. I suggest therapists to pay attention to their backgrounds; it needs to be fairly neutral, professional and unchanging from one session to the next to provide a sense of grounding and holding for clients. Seeing the client's background may give us materials for conversations that would not have been possible in the therapist's consulting room, for example, a piece of artwork that is on the client's wall. If clients or therapists choose a computer-generated background to hide their real background, there may be much transference and countertransference on what is to conceal, or a sense of rejection in some ways.

During the COVID-19 lockdowns, I'm pretty sure I met all my clients' pets. It can provide the therapy space with a bit of lightness and, sometimes, there may be a great opportunity for the animal to become a 'therapy pet'. Clients can find great soothing being around their pets, especially when revisiting painful memories or experiencing difficult emotions.

Accessibility and flexibility

Another general opportunity of online therapy is that it is more accessible for people. People with CSB don't only live in big cities where most specialist therapists work. Now, there are no more geographical blocks to accessing appropriate therapy; it can be more flexible. Without the travelling time to a therapist's office, clients can have their therapy at their lunch time or at more convenient times of day for them.

The black hole effect

Suler (1997) describes it as

> those moments on the internet when we initial some action and in return receive … nothing. Not even an error message. As if our intentions were completely gobbled up by some mysterious beast akin to those pits in outer space that swallow anything that comes their way, letting nothing escape.

Suler's words are meant to bring up a vivid picture of how some of us might feel when faced with a black hole. We can experience it if we send an e-mail to a client and never receive a response. Clients can easily disappear in cyberspace. Some of us call this phenomenon 'ghosting'. We may experience the Black Hole if there is a serious problem with connection and the computer suddenly goes blank. To avoid the Black Hole effect is to make sure therapists have another way of contacting the client, by phone for example. That way, if there is a break in connection in the middle of an intense conversation, therapists don't leave the client all by themselves with a blank screen for long. They can call the client straight away so that they have continued contact with them.

References

Suler, J. (1997). The black hole of cyberspace. [Available online]: http://users.rider.edu/~suler/psycyber/blackhole.html.

Suler, J. (2004). The psychology of cyberspace. [Available online]: http://www-usr.rider.edu/~suler/psycyber/disinhibit.html.

Part IV

Working with partners of people with CSB

Chapter 15

Assessment and formulation

Working with partners of people with CSB is very different work from working with clients with CSB. Some may come to therapy soon after a discovery, some may come years after the first discovery. It is not to say that someone who made a new discovery will necessarily be in more pain than someone who made the discovery long ago. Sometimes, it can be the other way around. After a recent discovery, some partners may be in shock or angry, but a few years later they may live in deep grief for the lost relationship.

Many clients will want to know '*why?*'. Therapists have to resist the urge to answer. We cannot tell clients that their partners might be having sexual compulsivity. We simply don't know. Some people will have repetitive affairs without compulsivity. The frame of the therapeutic space is to work with someone who is betrayed, not someone who is the 'victim of a sex addict'.

Some clients will be devastated in their initial consultation, others may be seductive in a way to reclaim their sexuality and self-esteem. Equally, in their home, some clients will want to be in a separate bedroom from their partners' whilst others will want to be sexual with them as soon as possible to keep them close.

Whether the partner decides to stay with the person with CSB and repair their relationship or not, there is an unavoidable major loss. Esther Perel (2017) asserts that a betrayal ends the relationship in its current form. It is then up to the couple to build a new relationship together or separately. In my initial consultation I acknowledge and validate the emotions and I conceptualise their presentations as a person who is in a long and complicated grief process.

Partners of people with CSB experience a wide range of emotions and responses after a discovery of betrayal. Their responses will depend on their psychological predispositions and external factors.

Psychological predispositions

1. **Attachment styles**. People will react to betrayal in various ways depending on their attachment styles.

2. **Self-esteem**. People with pre-existing poor self-esteem will struggle with emotional regulations more when faced with a betrayal.
3. **The quality of the connection with the partner with CSB.** Did they perceive their betraying partner as 'perfect' before the discovery? Were they genuinely happy in their marriage before the discovery? Did they ignore some red flags? Or were they already ambivalent about the relationship?
4. **Values.** Did the betrayal attack their core values to the extent of the impossibility of repair?
5. **Internalised messages from society and childhood**. Some people have strong conflicts between staying or leaving depending on some internalised messages they have, for example: '*You make your bed you lie in it*' or '*families should stay together at any cost*'. Or '*I can't leave whilst my children are still small*'.
6. **Personality traits.** People grieve according to their personality traits. The field of psychology identified the Big Five Personality Traits: openness to experience, conscientiousness, agreeableness, extraversion and neuroticism (Costa et al., 1992). People open to experience have high intellect levels and good imagination, which can complicate grief by imagining all sorts of scenarios or they become detectives. Conscientious people may become practical grievers. Extraverted people may grieve by reaching out to others, either their friends or a new lover. Agreeable people may want to put their partner's feelings first, understand their sexual compulsivity and try to make it work so that they can stay in the marriage. People with neuroticism usually have great difficulty in handling stress and find it hard to regulate their emotions. They tend to grieve in intense emotions of anger and sadness for a prolonged time.

External factors

1. The age of the children and co-parenting.
2. Financial situations.
3. The level of the betrayal. Not all betrayals are equal, and they are subjective.
4. How it was discovered. It is a different experience when someone admits their betrayal with taking responsibility, compared to someone discovering the betrayal when they get pubic crabs whilst their partner denies it.
5. How it was responded to. Did the betrayer blame the betrayed for their behaviours? Was there more gaslighting? Did the betrayer leave the relationship as soon as the discovery was made? Or did the betrayer show empathy, understanding, remorse, a willingness to repair the relationship?

6. The society in which they live. Some religious and cultural aspects of some people's life set-ups make it more difficult to have autonomy and to decide to leave the relationship because of shame, guilt, or status.

7. Stage of life. Some betrayed people may respond differently faced with the discovery of infidelity in relation to their stage of life. Are they at the beginning of a new career? Are they young? Is menopause looming? Do they have young children or are the children grown-up?

The grief process

When we think about grief, we automatically think of bereavement. It is easy to make a hierarchy of grief, someone dying is a bigger grief, or a more important grief, than someone being betrayed. It is important not to think of grief this way. Grief is not about who or what is lost. It is about the connection that we have with the person or object. Every grief is different because people grieve differently. There is not one way that is better than another way to grieve.

Here are examples of how some betrayed clients grieve:

1. Phillipa met Robert in her late twenties. It was love at first sight. She had had negative experiences with men before. She never felt loved by her father and her first boyfriend had cheated on her. When she met Robert, she thought he was different from all the others. She allowed herself to feel free and vulnerable with him. She perceived Robert as being the perfect '*Prince Charming*'. She lived in the fairy tale for twenty years, thinking she was so lucky to be in a great marriage with one of the few good men. Then, soon after her fiftieth birthday, and whilst starting the menopause process, she discovered that Robert had seen sex workers, about three times a year, through the entirety of their marriage. Her entire world collapsed. Her fairy tale was instantly destroyed. She felt shame for believing that good men existed. She felt stupid for being 'blind' to reality. She felt angry that Robert had let her believe in the Prince Charming that he clearly was not. She questioned the memories of the whole marriage, wondering if all of it had been a sham. She lost her entire story and beliefs of the last twenty years. Phillipa grieved multiple losses: her marriage, the fairy tale story that never was, her sense of self in that story, her tainted memories, the husband she thought she married, the love and peace she had felt. She was also grieving her 'womanhood' and changes in her sexuality because of the menopause. She lost any sense of grounding and roots.

2. Alan was very much in love with his girlfriend Amelia. They had been together for five years and they lived together. They were having serious conversations about buying a house together and having babies. In Alan's head, Amelia was the woman to settle down with for the rest of

his life. He was in his early thirties, with an expanding career that he enjoyed. Life was going his way, until one day; he sat in front of the communal computer and saw an e-mail account Amelia had forgotten to sign out of. In a space of a few minutes, Alan saw graphic images and texts of Amelia's sexual behaviours with multiple men. These occurrences happened several times a week with details of Amelia meeting them for sex. Alan was devastated. Life was not going his way after all. All of his future plans of buying a home and having a family was ruined instantly, and it took away his past five years. Just like Phillipa, Alan felt that his memories with Amelia were tainted. What was real and what wasn't? Having access to the e-mail account, Alan noticed that Amelia arranged to meet men for sex on his birthday. He had great memories of his last birthday, but now he wondered if she really was genuine then. Although Alan was in much pain and cried a lot, he was also a practical person. He said to me 'I'm a successful project manager and I will project manage this'. He did not lose his sense of self, he did not have any mutual finances, or dependents. The only thing they had together was a rented flat. He was sure about his boundaries and his values of monogamy. He decided to leave Amelia, grieve whilst connecting with friends. It took him a bit of time to recover from the graphic images and texts he saw, but because of helpful external factors, therapy was successful and relatively short-term. He gradually rebuilt a vision of his future without Amelia being part of the picture.

3. Ahman was in an open relationship with Mike for seven years. For Ahman, it was a very important relationship as it represented safety. He had suffered significant homophobic abuse from his family when he came out, losing his entire community. He thought it was worth it to be '*true to himself and his sexuality*'. He loved Mike and they both enjoyed including a third person in their sexual activities. They agreed on clear and specific rules: they only play together, no friendships with the third person, and condomless sex was reserved for the two of them only. Ahman was very happy with this relationship arrangement, he felt loved and accepted for the first time in his life. One Friday night, Mike didn't return home. Ahman was worried, it was out of character for Mike. He turned up on Saturday, in the late morning, looking ill. Mike confessed he had been in a Chemsex party and had a '*bad trip*'. This was devastating for Ahman. Mike had breached all of their important agreements that made him feel safe. He also felt great shame because he heard the voices of his homophobic family: '*that's what you get for being gay*', '*you will never find love*', '*love is not possible between two men*', '*gay men are sex maniacs*', and so on. Ahman asked Mike if it was the first time he did this. He asked the question without being prepared for the answer. Unfortunately, the answer was bad. Mike had done Chemsex

only a few times but he had been to sex clubs on a regular basis, not always using condoms, without Ahman's consent. Ahman was broken hearted. He no longer felt safe in his only refuge. He felt extra shame going to a sexual health clinic for a STI check. He found his friends being unhelpful too. They were all saying: *'leave him now, he's a bastard, get over him, find another man'*, and some were saying: *'that's what you get when you're in an open relationship'*. He felt criticised by his friends, at worst, and unsupported at best. Luckily, all STI tests came back negative. He didn't feel he had any space to grieve. He came to therapy to find a space of safety where he could take the time to grieve and to make sense of his story.

References

Costa et al. (1992). Normal personality assessment in clinical practice: the NEO personality inventory. *Psychological Assessment*, 4(1), 5–13.

Perel, E. (2017). *The state of affairs: rethinking infidelity*. London, UK: Yellow Kite.

Chapter 16

Grief

One of the best known grief models is the five stages of loss by Kubler-Ross and Kessler (2005):

1. Denial
2. Anger
3. Bargaining
4. Depression
5. Acceptance

Dr Kubler-Ross is clear that this model is not intended to describe a neat journey of stages, but a series of points that people may often revisit, or even experience all at once, or maybe not experience at all, as we adjust to a loss. Whilst it is helpful for some clients to identify their own language for their experience, it is helpful sometimes for them to see themselves in psychotherapeutic models.

Dr Lois Tonkins' model of grief, as discussed earlier in this book, does not define stages, but offers the perspective that we gradually grow around the grief. I think this perspective is useful to explain to clients because it is based on the idea that the loss, especially a major loss like a relationship or a marriage, may always be a part of us but that it eventually won't dominate how we live our lives. In essence, Dr Tonkin challenges the assumption that time heals all wounds. I find that talking to clients about it in that way takes away the pressure to stop feeling pain. With this model in mind, we can also avoid setting up an unrealistic goal that one day, they will not feel the pain and they can move on. The fact is that for some people, it is not possible. In times of special dates like anniversaries, people may feel sad, anger or a pinch in their heart when they connect to the loss, for the rest of their lives. It doesn't mean that they haven't grieved properly, it only means that they are human. The sign of healing is when the pain of the loss does not dominate someone's life. The image of growing around the grief has afforded Dr Tonkin the phrase of the 'fried egg model'. To me, it is similar to the Japanese pottery golden repair '*Kinsukuroi*'.

Clinical psychologists Stroebe and Schut developed a model of grief called the dual process model (2010). Their view of grief is that people oscillate between being 'loss-oriented', when they feel the unpleasant emotions of loss and 'restoration-oriented' when they think about other things, such as cooking, working, spending time with friends and so on. They say that it is with the oscillation that people eventually heal from the loss. I think this is a helpful model particularly for psychotherapists when they want to help clients who are in a complex and stuck grieving process. It is very much the same principle as multiple awareness. Helping clients move from different states and different awareness is a crucial part of processing difficult and painful emotions and cognition.

Julia Samuel (2020), a psychotherapist specialist in grief, guides us through the "*8 pillars of strength*", which I find is very helpful for clients to know whilst navigating grief:

1. Relationship with oneself. Accepting ourselves. Being kind and respectful to ourselves.
2. Relationship with others. Having strong friendships and connections with others. We need to make time to invest in those relationships.
3. Ways to manage emotions. Samuel proposes to be mindful of HALT (hungry, angry, lonely, tired) which are vulnerable times for making poor decisions.
4. Time. Being mindful of the present moment.
5. Mindbody. Regular exercise is good for the mind and the body.
6. Limits. Learning to say 'no' and being assertive.
7. Structure. Developing good habits with a routine in place helps feeling grounded.
8. Focusing. Practicing mindfulness.

The reconstruction of meaning

Neimeyer (2001) offers an important component of grieving which is meaning-making. People make their own understanding of the world by learning from their experiences. As we live life, we gather more evidence that informs some stories we tell ourselves about the world and where we stand in it. When a major loss comes, those stories, which are often part of our core beliefs, may be deeply shaken. People might feel like nothing makes sense anymore. For example, some people may have lived a life so far with assumptions like:

'*If I'm a good citizen, good things will happen to me*'
'*If I follow the rules of society, I will be rewarded*'
'*The world is a fair place, you get back what you put in*'
'*If I'm a good partner, my marriage will be great*'

For many people, such assumptions are the strong building blocks of their understanding of the world and life. Facing a major intimate betrayal can suddenly destroy these building blocks, leaving clients feeling emotionally 'homeless'. The betrayal, the loss and the grief require clients to find a way to build a new meaning, a new story for themselves.

Some clients who reached the stage of meaning-making often describe gratitude for the betrayal and the loss because it got them to change for the best. When Phillipa learnt she could live in a world where she could have her own sense of self rather than relying on someone else being her 'rock' was life-changing for her. Alan took the opportunity to feel proud of himself for dealing with his loss in his pragmatic ways and making the right decisions for himself. It reinforced his secure attachment style as his self-worth was not destroyed by the betrayal. Ahman learnt that being with Mike was not his punishment for being gay. He became more aware of self-love and not blaming himself for the actions of another. He became more comfortable living in a world where '*shit happens even when you're a good boyfriend*'. He challenged his internalised homo-negativity inherited from his parents.

Disenfranchised grief

Esther Perel (2017) reminds us that when we say 'partner' it may also refer to the illegitimate person, as they, too, are partners of the person with CSB. Some people with sexual compulsivity build connections and relationships with other people outside of their primary relationship. When the primary partner makes the discovery, the person with CSB will often suddenly stop all other relationships, permanently or temporarily, in an attempt to save their relationship. This leaves this other partner(s) grieving too as there is a loss of connection that can be as distressing and as intensely emotional as primary partners feel. Often, people who are 'the third partner' will experience their grief in silence, with a shaming sense that they're not allowed to feel the grief. Friends can be unsympathetic saying: '*why did you think he was going to leave his wife?*', '*you got yourself in a mess*', and so on. Societal messages dismiss the validity of the grief for the 'third partner'. This is what we call Disenfranchised Grief. The shame and the disenfranchised grief may be a reason for 'the third partner' to seek therapy. As psychotherapists, we must be as empathic and validating with this population as we are with primary partners. Disenfranchised grief can quickly become complex.

Disenfranchised grief also happens when the discovery of CSB takes place after the death of the primary partner (Neves, 2018). This makes for confusing grieving. Can the surviving partner grieve the loss of the partner they thought they shared their lives with? Should they grieve the loss of the meaning of their relationship where there will be no possibility to find answers? It is such a shaming experience that surviving partners usually grieve the betrayal-related loss in silence whilst maintaining a public loss of what is now felt as a lie.

Complex grief diagnosis

The most recent versions of official diagnostic guidelines include a diagnosis of '*Prolonged Grief Disorder*' in the ICD-11 and '*Persistent Complex Bereavement Disorder*' in the DSM-5.

ICD11: Prolonged grief disorder

Guidelines for this diagnosis include the occurrence of a '*persistent and pervasive grief response characterised by longing for the deceased or persistent preoccupation with the deceased accompanied by intense emotional pain (e.g. sadness, guilt, anger, denial, blame, difficulty accepting the death, feeling one has lost a part of one's self, an inability to experience positive mood, emotional numbness, difficulty in engaging with social or other activities)*'.

DSM-5: Persistent complex bereavement disorder (PCBD)

This refers to as '*severe and persistent grief and mourning reaction*' in '*Other Specified Trauma- and Stressor-Related Disorders*' (p. 289).

Although the diagnosis of complex grief is mostly understood in the context of loss by death, these symptoms are observed in people grieving other losses, included loss of relationship, even with clients who decide to stay with the partner who betrayed them. The terms '*Complicated Grief*' and '*Traumatic Grief*' are also used for people who suffer with extreme grief responses over prolonged periods of time.

References

DSM-5. *Diagnostic and statistical manual of mental disorders*, 5th ed. Philadelphia, PA: American Psychiatric Association.

ICD-11. *International classification of disease*. 11th revision. World Health Organisation. [Available online]: https://icd.who.int/en.

Kubler-Ross, E. and Kessler, D. (2005). *On grief and grieving: finding the meaning of grief through the five stages of loss*. London: Simon & Schuster UK.

Neimeyer, R.A. (2001). *Meaning reconstruction and the experience of loss*. Washington, DC: American Psychological Association.

Neves, S. (2018). Disenfranchised grief. *BACP Private Practice Journal* (December), 9–11.

Perel, E. (2017). *The state of affairs: rethinking infidelity*. London: Yellow Kite.

Samuel, J. (2020). *This too shall pass*. London: Penguin Life.

Stroebe, M. and Schut, H. (2010). *The dual process model of coping with bereavement: a decade on*. Omega, 61(4), 273–289.

Tonkin, L., *Growing around grief*. [Available online]: http://www.loistonkin.com/growing-around-grief.html.

Chapter 17

Trauma

Many partners of people with CSB describe feeling traumatised after the discovery of hidden sexual behaviours. When someone discovers a long history of hidden sexual behaviours spanning many years, or throughout their marriage, the impact can be traumatising when:

1. The betrayed feels that their entire relationship was a lie.
2. The betrayal causes a re-evaluation of their whole life.
3. They experience a rupture in their sense of who they thought they were in a relationship with 'who is this person?'.
4. They realise how much time their betraying partner has spent away from them to be with others in secret.
5. They realise how much money their partner has spent on the CSB.
6. They feel exploited – the betrayed partner did not get to choose or make decisions about their relationship, their lives, their here and now and their future as they did not have all of the information.
7. Gaslighting or abuse has been a feature of their partner's behaviour.
8. Their world view is shattered – 'I thought people were good and kind', 'I'm a nice person and bad things don't happen if you are nice'.

Gaslighting

Gaslighting is a term borrowed from the 1944 film *Gaslight*. The premise of the film is a husband protecting a secret by making his wife think she is going insane. Gaslighting is now a popular term to describe such behaviours in relationships. Gaslighting is an abusive behaviour because it is coercive and requires a high level of psychological manipulation. Gaslighting is not the same as being lied to. Many people lie for different reasons. Some lie to protect themselves or protect their partner from hurt. Some lie to avoid conflicts or to hide a behaviour that they don't really want to stop. Although it may be hard to believe, most people who lie still love and respect their partner in some way. However, gaslighting is an abusive behaviour that goes beyond lying, and is beyond love and respect.

The intention of gaslighting is to make someone think they're crazy, so it takes much resentment and contempt from the gaslighter to do that and to continue doing it. Gaslighting may occur if, for example, a betrayed person has evidence of their betraying partner's breach of boundaries and the partner's response is:

You're overreacting.
You're upset over nothing.
I didn't do it.
You must be confused again.
Just calm down.
You're so dramatic.
Why are you so defensive?
I never did it.
What are you talking about?
It's your fault.
You twist things.
You're so sensitive.
Stop imagining things.
It's not a big deal.
You're remembering things wrong.
There's always something up with you.
You're always unhappy about something.
You're mentally ill.
You should get help, you're crazy.

Please remember that if these things are said as a one-off defence after being caught lying or cheating, it wouldn't constitute gaslighting. Gaslighting is when it is a persistent intention to twist the person's reality to make them doubt their own mind, for the gain of the gaslighter.

Relational trauma

Relational trauma is defined as being intentionally hurt by someone with whom there is a loving bond. Non-consensual non-monogamy can be a relational trauma.

Working with partners of CSB who identify as being traumatised is a delicate area because, on one hand, we must validate their traumatising experience; on the other hand, it is important not to collude with sex-negativity such as:

1. *'I'm traumatised because my partner watched pornography'* (unless watching pornography was previously discussed as unacceptable due to strong values – most of the time, it is not discussed explicitly).

2. *'I'm traumatised because my partner has wandering eyes'*.
3. *'I'm traumatised because my partner objectifies women'*.
4. *'I'm traumatised because my partner has sexual fantasies about other people'*.
5. *'I'm traumatised because my partner wears stockings or has a leather fetish'*.

These do not meet the traditional definitions of trauma nor the definition of relational trauma. However, we must still validate the client's emotions, but instead of colluding with it, we can enquire further and be curious as to why they experience it as trauma. We can help clients by normalising both: their partner's fetish is not an attack on them, however, being lied to hurts.

Exploring these issues carefully and with empathy can open the space for clients to understand themselves better. For example, it may be that they never thought about what sexual fantasies really are. I find that normalising what people don't know about sexology can help clients see their partner's erotic in a different light, and reduces anxiety.

I help clients identify what they're really upset about. Are they upset that their partner watches pornography? Or are they upset that they watch it in secret? Are they upset they've been lied to? Are they upset their partner watches people who look different from them? Are they upset because they feel insecure? It is helpful for clients to figure out what their wound is as they are often confused; intense emotions come without a clear story.

Polygraph: a harmful practice to never do in the context of CSB

Over the years, I have heard of 'sex addiction' therapists using a polygraph test on their clients with CSB to facilitate a process of full disclosure with their partners. I urge all my readers to never even think of using a polygraph. There are companies out there who will happily sell you their polygraph service. Do not do it.

Psychotherapy is not the court of law. Psychotherapy to treat compulsive sexual behaviours is not about *'coming clean'* and it is certainly not about criminal behaviours. Submitting a client with compulsive sexual behaviours to a polygraph sends a harmful psychological message: *'You're a bad person'*, *'you're a criminal'*, *'you cannot be trusted'*, reinforcing clients' existing negative core beliefs, which therapy should attempt to treat. Doing a polygraph is counter-therapeutic, and counter-productive in every way imaginable.

Reference

Gaslight. (1944). Film starring Charles Boyer and Ingrid Bergman. Director: George Cukor. Turner Entertainment and Warner Bros Entertainment. DVD. Available on Amazon.co.uk.

Chapter 18

Clinical interventions: Phase 1

My three-phase treatment protocol can also be used when treating partners of people with CSB:

Phase 1: regulation
Phase 2: processing
Phase 3: reconstruction

Phase 1: regulation

Partners are likely to come to their initial consultation in a crisis. They will be upset, angry and ashamed. Some can feel resentful to be speaking to a therapist. I often hear: 'why am I sitting here? It's all his/her problem! Nothing to do with me!' They may be right, but I help partners reframe their thoughts about that: they are not in therapy to help stop the sexual compulsivity, they are in therapy because they have a broken heart and are in grief. I think it is important to reframe early, because therapy often goes wrong when there is too much emphasis on their partner's sexual compulsivity, and what they can do to stop it from happening again.

Because they will be upset, it is crucial to help clients with emotional regulation. They will need to regulate their emotions for different circumstances:

1   Emotional regulation when they are triggered.
2   Emotional regulation when they feel the pain of grief.
3   Emotional regulation for shame reduction.
4   Emotional regulation when engaging with their betraying partner.

Emotional regulation when they are triggered

Triggers can happen in various ways. The more clients know about the details of the sexual compulsivity behaviours of their partner, the more they will have triggers. With some people, these triggers can be so intense that they can impair their life.

Maria always wanted children but she was unable to have any because of medical reasons. She grieved the impossibility of having children years ago. She was happy in her marriage with Fabio until she discovered that he had multiple affairs with women who were mothers. Since the discovery, Maria was intensely triggered with big waves of uncontrollable emotion each time she saw women with children in the streets, which would be almost daily. It made her life difficult to live. Mark found out that his partner Drew engaged in frequent sex parties with a neighbour. He found it unbearable to live in the same street, seeing the neighbour's house every day. David discovered that his wife Julie had multiple sex encounters with young, muscle-bound footballer types, whilst he was ageing and considered himself as *'having a beer belly'*. Each time he saw an athletic man in the street or on television, he would be triggered with enormous sadness and anger at his body.

Triggers are embedded in somatic markers that relate to our five senses (visual, scent, sound, touch and taste) and also stories or themes.

The triggers are activated when clients encounter a somatic marker and lose their grounding in that moment. For example, Maria might not have had such a trigger if the fertility theme wasn't sensitive for her. Mark might have found it easier to manage his emotions if Drew chose to have sex parties further away rather than on his doorstep. David might have been able to regulate his emotions better if he felt more confident about his body and didn't compare himself with athletic young men. I don't mean to say that their hurt is related to their sensitivity. Even someone with the best self-esteem would be hurt at the discovery of betrayal, but for some who have unmanageable triggers, it is often to do with their own wounds being activated.

The dual process concept of grief by Stroebe and Schut (2010) is a key emotional regulation strategy for desensitising triggers, helping clients to pendulate between the hurt of the wound and an orientation of self-care, back and forth.

> *Fabio betrayed me with mothers. I am furious about that. And I know that I am not defective.*
> *I think Drew is a disrespectful lazy man for choosing to cheat on me across the road. And it does not make me a naïve, stupid person. I can still walk down the street knowing that I have been a good partner.*
> *Although Julie likes to have sex with athletic men, it doesn't make me any less sexy. Many women like a 'beer belly', it is a matter of preference.*

Some CBT enquiries can be helpful to address negative cognitions:

Do you believe this all the time?
Would you say the same things to a friend who was going through the same problems?
What are you good at?
What do you do well?
Is it a useful thought/belief?
If not, might there be a more useful thought to have?
What would happen if you didn't let this trigger control your thoughts and feelings?

Of course, the dual process is difficult, especially at the beginning of therapy. Not all clients are ready to do this work. If there is unwillingness, it may be an indication that clients need to express their pain of grief first, without the pressure of changing it.

Emotional regulation when they feel the pain of grief

The best intervention to help clients regulate their emotions with grief is the therapeutic relationship and the therapist's witnessing of the client's pain. Allowing a space where clients can express themselves freely is an important initial step to therapy. The psychotherapist will need to use their clinical judgement as to when to address some issues and when to simply hold the space for them. Some clients will express their grief mostly with anger and call their partners all kind of insults, and blame them and say common things like: '*I wish he'd die, it would have been less painful!*', '*I hope she got an STD!*' or '*I want to cut his dick off'* and so on. In the initial stages, it may be beneficial for the therapist to hold the proverbial bucket for clients to vomit their anger without challenging them. However, an absence of challenge doesn't mean collusion. There are many facial expressions, body languages and sounds the therapist can make to communicate collusion in those moments. We must be careful not to do so. When the time is right, the therapist can then challenge some of these thoughts: validating their grief, and anger but helping clients stay with their own values of integrity.

Are you the kind of person who wishes serious harm to your partner, even after doing what he did? Most clients will say 'no'.

Some clients express their grief mostly with sadness. The discovery of the enormous betrayal can destabilise a client into feeling '*destroyed*'. They live in a fog, they cannot recognise any reality, and they are in deep sadness. Allowing space and offering our full presence for clients to feel without any pressure to fix is essential and healing. With some people, the devastation of the betrayal is so intense that it goes beyond words. Sitting with clients in silence, with our full presence, has a healing power that is often under-rated in psychotherapy. A 'talking therapy' needs silence sometimes.

Some clients may express their grief with denial, or shall we say, unrealistic expectations. They want their relationship and their life to be back to what it was overnight. They want to stop feeling hurt immediately. They may have unrealistic expectations of the therapist, thinking we should have a magic wand to take the pain away. They have unrealistic expectations or demands of their partner as an attempt to stop the pain.

> *You will stop watching porn and masturbating straight away.*
> *You will tell me everything you fantasise about.*
> *You will always leave work on time.*
> *You will give me access to your phone whenever I want it.*
> *You will give me full control of our finances.*
> *I will never have sex with you again and you will not masturbate or watch porn ever again.*
> *You will not look at other people in the streets, only me.*
> *You will not have sexual fantasies again.*
> *You will have to be sorry for the rest of your life.*

It is the psychotherapist's uncomfortable task to tell such clients that these thoughts, wishes or demands are unrealistic. Many of these unrealistic expectations will make the problems worse and none of it will take their pain away. Instead, psychotherapists can negotiate with clients that the first step is allowing the grieving process to happen, and it takes time.

There are few resources or support for partners of people with CSB. They often have to resort to 12-step type meetings like *S-Anon*, which I don't recommend (as you know by now). These meetings can fuel anger and demonise normative sexual behaviours. They are usually populated by a great majority of women, which can encourage and normalise misandry. Partners of people with CSB usually come to see me after feeling stuck in one of these meetings because they are encouraged to stay with a label of '*victim*', which becomes unhelpful over time. The best support outside of therapy that clients can hope for is a good non-judgmental friend. Not everybody is lucky enough to have one of them, especially in long-term relationships when good friends are often mutual friends with their partner with CSB. In the absence of the possibility to connect with friends, I think clients do well with focusing on a passionate engagement of their choice.

Emotional regulation for shame reduction

I think the process of self-compassion discussed in Part 3 is one of the best methods to soothe shame. In practical terms, self-compassion to reduce shame sounds something like that:

1   *I feel bad for myself.*
2   *My feeling bad is my shame.*
3   *I'm going to take a moment and breathe through this feeling.*
4   *I'm feeling the shame and I accept myself too.*
5   *Even though I feel shame I can love myself. Client can put a warm hand on the part of the body that is soothing, the chest or forehead for example, gently. 'I am a human being worthy of love'.*
6   *Everybody feels bad sometimes. It is a human experience to have unpleasant feelings sometimes. Everybody has these moments.*

This is only meant to be a guide, the process will be slightly different, depending on the clients and the situations.

Psycho-education

As part of psycho-education, there are some 'Dos' and 'Don'ts' that you can suggest to clients. Shame is often fed by myths and stories we make up. All good information based on reality can help reduce shame a little.

Do's

1   Remember their rights as a human being.
2   Check values.
3   Challenge their own thoughts if they only stay in the relationship for the children.
4   Continue to engage in therapy .
5   Retain the choice to stay or leave the relationship, make regular evaluations.
6   Seek legal advice if they're married or have a joint business together. Seeking legal advice doesn't mean they're making the decision to divorce, it means they're gathering all the information they need to help them with making a decision.
7   Normalise all the range of emotions.
8   Say 'no' to others to say 'yes' to themselves.
9   Be prepared that the relationship will never be the same again.
10 If they want to stay in the relationship, do be prepared that they will need to make changes too.

Don'ts

1   Become a detective. Clients often come to therapy having been a detective already. I validate their detective ability and I also tell them that they have done enough detective work and they don't need to do any more.
2   Look for more details. They know enough. Details will only create more negative somatic markers and more triggers.

3   Lean on their children for their emotional regulation.
4   Look for a rescuer.
5   Become abusive – Being betrayed is not a green card to be abusive.
6   Make threats – *'I will destroy your career', 'I will take the children away'* – this is also abusive.
7   Make drastic decisions for at least six months after the discovery to give themselves plenty of space.
8   Think that the relationship will 'get back to normal'.
9   Think only their partner has to make changes.

Emotional regulation when engaging with their partner

Boundaries

Although I don't recommend clients prescribing what their partner should do with their sex lives or their fantasies, I do recommend that my clients know about their own boundaries and express them clearly to their partner. Often, when it is monogamy that has been breached, I ask my client how monogamy was defined and discussed when they first met. I hear most of the time that it had never been discussed because they assumed that monogamy meant just one thing. But monogamy can be defined in different ways: for some couples sexting and flirting with others is ok, whilst it is unacceptable for other couples, for example. Whether the original arrangement was a monogamous or a polyamorous one, the client's relational values might have changed temporarily as a result of the betrayal. Therapists can help clients decide what they need to happen in the relationship in the here-and-now so that they can begin to heal. The Traffic Light Exercise is helpful for clients to figure out their boundaries in details.

Green: what they need to happen in the relationship that is realistic.
Amber: what needs to be on hold or up for discussion.
Red: what must not happen in the relationship that is realistic.

Many clients will be confused about what they want and need at the aftermath of the discovery of betrayal. Some say: *'I don't know anymore what a relationship should be like'*. As a guide to help clients understand what they want for themselves, I draw on the work of Dr Sue Johnson's *'Hold Me Tight'*. Her A.R.E. conversations can produce some profound shifts in clients' thinking.

A – *Accessibility: Can I reach you?*
R – *Responsiveness: Can I rely on you to respond to me emotionally?*
E – *Engagement: Do I know you will value me and stay close? (2008, pp. 49–50).*

I think accessibility, responsiveness and engagement, are useful themes to think about relationships in more depth. I ask clients to think about them as their guide to make requests for change for their partner with CSB, but also a frame for what to look for in their future relationship, whether it is with their current partner or a new one. These reflections can provide ideas on what they want in their Green, Amber and Red sections of their Traffic Light. Once they are sure about their boundaries, the psychotherapist can help clients find their way to express these to their partner in a useful manner.

The Traffic Light exercise and boundaries should be up for review on a regular basis because they can change over time when there is or isn't progress in their relationships. However, clients have to be clear to keep re-asserting boundaries if they get breached again.

Staying or leaving?

Whilst it is an easy decision for some to make, it is a tormenting one for many. Although clients may report feeling broken hearted and deeply hurt, it doesn't always switch off love. I offer clients a space to discuss honestly some of the reasons why they want to stay in the relationship. It may be because they are hopeful that the relationship will improve. Or they might not want to lose their partner's family with whom they created loving bonds. They might be economically dependent on their partner. Perhaps they are afraid of being alone. For some, they are staying in order to prevent their partner from having a new sexual partner, or they don't want to be intimate with anyone else. It is worth reminding clients that they have a right to change their mind and they might fluctuate a lot between wanting to stay and wanting to leave. It is ok to be in the in-between space for a while.

How to speak to children

For couples who have children, protecting them against the chaos of the discovery of betrayal and its aftermath is a central concern that partners of people with CSB bring to the consulting room. It is the psychotherapist's role working with such clients to help them navigate how they will talk to children about it. Firstly, I say that it is never helpful to say: '*your father/ mother is a sex addict*'. It is loaded in shame and pathology, it will be humiliating to the person with CSB and the children will feel disgusted by it, which is not a good thing. Secondly, whether the children or still minors or not, it is never a good idea to lean on them for safety, love and care or, worse, as a confidant. It is also not appropriate to tell them about their private sex life or the one of their partners. Even adult children don't want to hear it. Thirdly, I offer my clients some broad guidelines:

1   Your children probably know something is going on. They can pick things up more than you want to imagine. It is not a good idea to ignore the obvious as children will feel lied to. But it is not appropriate to tell them the gritty details.
2   They want to be reassured that they won't be abandoned.
3   They want to be reassured that both parents will continue to love them.
4   They want to know it is not their fault that their parents have problems.
5   They want to know in advance if one of the parents will move out so that they can get prepared for the change.
6   They want to know what will happen to them if there is a divorce.

References

Johnson, S. (2008). *Hold Me Tight*. London, UK: Piatkus.

S-Anon. [Available Online]: https://sanon.org.

Stroebe, M. and Schut, H. (2010). The dual process model of coping with bereavement: a decade on. *Omega*, 61(4), 273–289.

Chapter 19

Clinical interventions: Phase 2

Phase 2: reprocessing

If clients engage well with the first phase of emotional regulation, they will get a sense of some control back and self-reliance. It may be all they need to support themselves with their grief process. Having a weekly contact with their psychotherapist whom they trust and who knows the whole story is healing in itself. The weekly point of contact may serve as a regular check in of their emotions and thoughts, a reminder to keep to their self-care and boundaries and help them meet any difficult emotions they have regarding their partner and the relationship. There isn't always a need for reprocessing for this client group.

However, for some clients, the betrayal will have re-opened past wounds. These clients are not only hurt by the here-and-now betrayal, they are re-acting to something older, often an unresolved trauma or childhood issues. For these clients, the reprocessing phase is the next step. The betrayal is an opportunity to treat other dormant trauma. This is when therapy is no longer about their partner cheating, but about them.

Depending on the client's story, psychotherapists can use all of their traditional therapeutic skills: Gestalt, Attachment-based psychotherapy, psychodynamic psychotherapy, Transactional Analysis, CBT, ACT, and, of course, trauma therapy as discussed in Part 3.

Some clients will identify some unhelpful core beliefs about sex and relationship. For example, a typical one for women is: '*you make your bed you lie in it*', which will be a block for them to assert their boundaries and make a conscious decision about what they want to do with their relationship. For men, it may be: '*being cheated on means you're a lesser man*'.

Samantha discovered her husband breached their monogamous agreement by having sex with multiple sex workers over many years. When she confronted her husband about it, he reacted in an abusive way, blaming her for his behaviours, telling her he didn't love her and left the house that same day, never to return. The hurt of the betrayal and the brutal way in which her husband reacted reminded her of being abandoned by her father overnight in childhood. Although the story is very different, the theme is the same; not being loved and being left overnight. Samantha's relationship with her husband was her way of feeling loved and fending off her childhood wounds. When her relationship was taken away so suddenly, she lost her sense of self, she felt both the intense hurt of the here-and-now betrayal and the childhood wound re-opened and hurt again, twice as much. Samantha could not function in her life, she had to take time off work, and she fell into a severe depression for a while. She didn't want a divorce when her husband asked for it because she could not cope with that ultimate loss. The more she stalled with the divorce, the more her husband became psychologically abusive to her. She struggled to keep boundaries in place because she preferred to sustain the abuse than to have him out of her life completely, as she still struggled with the wounds her father inflicted on her. It took many sessions to support Samantha through the Phase 1 of emotional regulation. When her father left, nothing was ever discussed, she felt that she didn't have space to talk about her feelings then. The consulting room was the first place where she could do so. She was clearer with her boundaries doing the Traffic Light exercise and she was now aware that she did not want to let go of the marriage because she didn't want to be intimate with anyone else. At that point, Samantha was ready for Phase 2. I helped her get in touch with her internal script: '*I am not good enough on my own*', '*I need to sexually please a man to get him to stay*', '*if I don't it means my father was right to leave me all along*'. She engaged well in trauma therapy to reprocess her childhood wounds from her father. I used Chairwork to address her young self which was a moving self-reparenting piece. She engaged well with visualisation to enhance her renewed self-esteem. She then gained a new perspective on her marriage and her separation. She was now ready to let go of her husband and, for the first time in her adult life, she was ready to be a single woman.

Chapter 20

Clinical interventions: Phase 3

Reconstruction: a new understanding of the world

Clients can piece together their story, with the new meaning they made about themselves. Even for clients who may not need much of Phase 2, they often benefit from Phase 3 because all betrayals are a major loss and grief. This is when I might suggest clients re-visit their Traffic Lights exercise and check what they want to include for the vision of their new sex and relationship life.

Forgiveness

I think it is unfair when therapists put the pressure on their clients to forgive their partner in order to move on. I don't agree with it. The idea of the need to forgive has a taste of moral religiosity for me. Some betraying sexual behaviours can be so unacceptable for our clients, attacking and wounding such a core part of their self, that sometimes forgiveness is absolutely not possible, nor should it be. Encouraging a client to somehow find forgiveness can make a client feel defective, again. However, the therapist can help clients be self-compassionate for not being able to forgive.

Repairing the relationship

Perel (2017) writes

> In my work I have identified three basic post-infidelity outcomes for couples who choose to stay together (with thanks to Helen Fisher for the typology): those who get stuck in the past (the sufferers); those who pull themselves up by the bootstraps and let it go (the builders); and those who rise above the ashes and create a better union (the explorers) (p. 292).

I couldn't agree more with this statement. Some people, the "sufferers", find a hidden gain at being in a perpetual disagreement, disappointment and anger, where their relationship is defined by their differences and resentment rather than their similarities and kindness. Often, these are people who grew up in similar households. As Perel describes it so vividly: *"they are sharing a cell in marital prison"*. The *"builders"* are those who care about each other and want to uphold their original relationship commitment, so they carry on as normal without making significant changes. Some may choose to believe of the possibility to erase that inconvenient part of their story, although rather than erasing it, they put it in a box out of sight, in the attic. The *"explorers"* are the ones for whom the betrayal becomes an opportunity for transforming their relationship. They are able to find the gold nuggets through the intense pain and make some *'kinsukuroi'*.

I use the analogy of planets to represent a relationship (this is because of my love of cosmology). I ask my clients what kind of planet they want to live in. One that is frozen, inhospitable, no places for growth. One that is dusty, not as bad as the frozen one, but not comfortable either, yet they can make do with a tent. Or are they up for living in a flourishing world, full of growth, colours and possibilities?

The icy planet

Four years after the last betrayal, Janet constantly reminded Phil of his cheating. She told him that she would never be happy for the rest of her life as he had taken the joy away from her. She insulted him with *'you're sick'* and a *'you're a sex addict'* at every opportunity, each time there was a pretty actress on television, for example. She withdrew completely from him and expected him to be non-sexual. His only sexual outlet was to watch pornography and masturbate in secret.

The dusty planet

Nick loved Erin. They were high school sweethearts. He was so attached to her that he had decided to brush Erin's strings of sexual betrayal under the carpet. Erin vowed to him that she had changed now and she committed to monogamy again and wanted to finally settle down with Nick and start a family. Nick didn't want his family and friends to think bad of Erin nor did he want others to perceive their marriage as less than perfect. They decided to let Erin's betrayal go and continue on the path that they had started before the betrayal. They avoided talking about any event that might remind them of the betrayal.

The flourishing planet

Declan loves Guy despite his multiple betrayals with anonymous sex in saunas for several years. After all the hurt, they both explored openly if they wanted to be monogamous or not. Guy did his therapeutic work to heal his own childhood trauma. Declan did his therapeutic work to figure out why and how he chose Guy, why he wanted to stay with him and what he would need to change for himself. Declan and Guy decided to return to the drawing board with their mutual new understanding, being clear about their principles of sexual health. They both consciously decided to stay in monogamy and with an open and continual erotic conversation, they both chose to be more honest with themselves and each other about their shared vision and mutual pleasure. They were open to take on the challenge of being in radical acceptance of each other. Their planet post-betrayal looked more flourishing and colourful; completely different from the one they started their relationship in.

Radical acceptance

Radical acceptance is the essential ingredient for a flourishing relationship planet. It requires what we call 'differentiation' (Bader and Pearson, 2012); how we can be in meaningful relationships and stand on our own two feet at the same time. My definition of radical acceptance is the following:

1   One human being cannot meet all of your needs.
2   Accept what you can't change.
3   Empower yourself to make the changes that can be made.
4   Make the changes yourself before requesting your partner to change. If you make some changes yourself, you will change the system, and therefore your partner can respond to the system change.
5   Empower yourself to stand as an independent and self-reliant person and meet your partner in the third space. The relationship is the third space. Be mindful that each decision you make will have an impact on your partner. When you need to meet your needs, you need to consider your partner with kindness, but you must not ignore your needs for the sake of your partner, trusting that the relationship is robust enough to withstand those difficult conversations and disappointment.
6   Allow your partner to have needs that are outside of the relationship: time on their own, separate hobbies and a private part of their erotic mind. As long as there are enough shared values, shared vision and shared interests, it can actually be very good for people to have a hobby where partners are not included.

Separating

Meg-John Barker gives us an opportunity to re-think the traditional binary story of break-up, when there needs to be *"good guys and bad guys"*. Instead, they encourage us to think beyond the rules, into embracing uncertainty:

We want to find something sure and certain to cling to: an anchor in the storm. Particularly we want reassurance that we're okay, given our underlying fear that we might not be. Ironically, grasping the anchor is what often pulls us under, whereas allowing ourselves to float free on an ocean of multiple possibilities can see us to calmer waters. We need to hold onto many stories, even when they might be contradiction, rather than searching for one simple truth (2018, p. 255).

When clients decide to separate from their betraying partners, therapists can guide some conversations about keeping their multiple stories intact for themselves. Although their spouse cheated, they can still keep and cherish some good memories they had together. Even when clients realise that they have been cheated on doesn't mean that they weren't loved by their partner. Although they may not want to be with their partner any longer doesn't mean they are bad people. Some people who betray others can also be good human beings in other ways. Separating from their partner whilst humanising them is the best balanced position to step out of the relationship with love and kindness.

The art of rest

When a relationship is in upheaval, when there are broken hearts, when there is much grief and loss, when past trauma re-surface, there are opportunities for clients to re-evaluate their lives as a whole in an attempt to bring more balance. I find that one of the most overlooked behaviours that creates good balance is resting. In a world where we place high value in speedy achievements and success, we have to remind ourselves that we need to rest. It sounds simple, yet it doesn't come naturally to some people. Hammond (2019) reminds us that there are many ways we can rest, most of them are solitary ways, a time of respite and quiet for ourselves, whether it is watching television, daydreaming, a good walk or doing nothing in particular.

References

Bader, E. and Pearson, P.T. (2012). *In quest of the mythical mate: a developmental approach to diagnosis and treatment in couples therapy*. Abingdon, UK: Routledge.

Barker, M.J. (2018). *Rewriting the rules*, 2nd ed. Abingdon, UK: Routledge.

Hammond, C. (2019). *The art of rest: how to find respite in the modern age*. Edinburgh, UK: Canongate Books.

Perel, E. (2017). *The state of affairs: rethinking infidelity*. London, UK: Yellow Kite.

Conclusion

Sexual compulsivity causes tremendous chaos not only in people's lives, but in their partners' as well. The condition sits tightly in all the neighbourhoods of a person's psyche, feeds in shame and thrives in the dissonance of a person's sense of self. The less awareness people have about their Erotic Template, the stronger the compulsivity. The treatment of compulsive sex isn't merely about stopping sexual behaviours. Equipped with sex-positivity and a wide range of psychotherapy modalities, we can help clients look at the disturbances underneath their sexual compulsivity, visit the parts of their selves that are infected with shame and trauma, and resolve these problems. Psychotherapy for sexual compulsivity is the golden repair for a profound shift into the new meaning of a person's existence.

Index